EVERYDAY ANTI-INFLAMMATORY DIET COOKBOOK

120 Simple Recipes to Reduce Inflammation, Boost Immunity, and Feel Your Best

Jennifer Lindsey

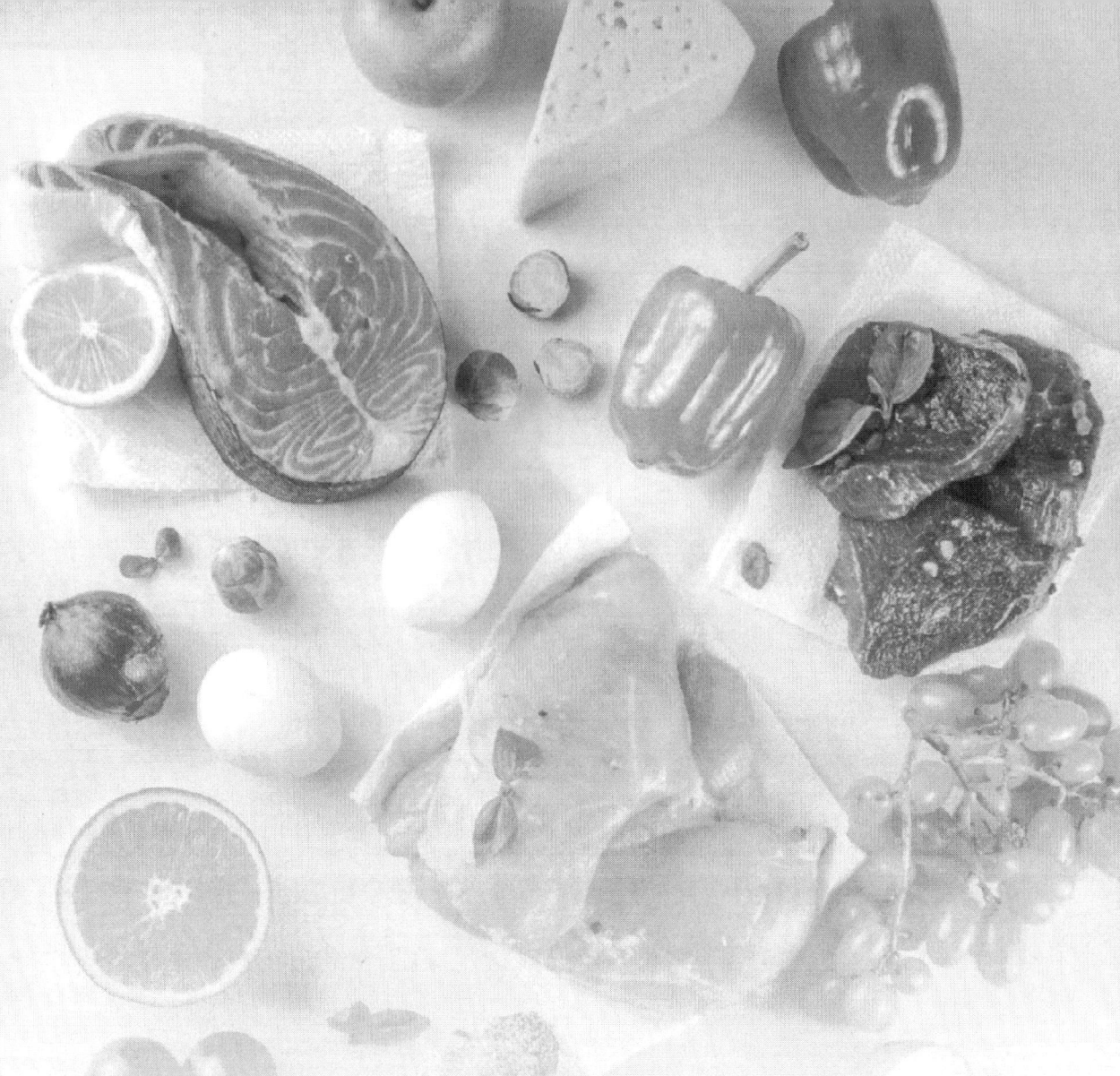

Copyright © 2024 - Jennifer Lindsey - All rights reserved.
The content within this book may not be reproduced, duplicated, or transmitted without direct written permission from the author or the publisher. Under no circumstances will any blame or legal responsibility be held against the publisher, or author, for any damages, reparation, or monetary loss due to the information contained within this book, either directly or indirectly.

Legal Notice:
This book is copyright protected. It is only for personal use. You cannot amend, distribute, sell, use, quote, or paraphrase any part of the content within this book, without the consent of the author or publisher.

Disclaimer Notice:
Please note the information contained within this document is for educational and entertainment purposes only. All effort has been expended to present accurate, up-to-date, reliable, and complete information. No warranties of any kind are declared or implied. Readers acknowledge that the author is not engaged in the rendering of legal, !nancial, medical, or professional advice. The content within this book has been derived from various sources. Please consult a licensed professional before attempting any techniques outlined in this book.

By reading this document, the reader agrees that under no circumstances is the author responsible for any losses, direct or indirect, that are incurred as a result of the use of the information contained within this document, including, but not limited to, errors, omissions, or inaccuracies.

INTRODUCTION

Welcome to Everyday Anti-Inflammatory Diet Cookbook: 100 Simple Recipes to Reduce Inflammation, Boost Immunity, and Feel Your Best. This book is your companion on a journey to better health through the power of food. It's designed to help you nourish your body, reduce chronic inflammation, and enjoy the process of cooking and eating meals that fuel your well-being.

Inflammation is the body's natural defense mechanism, but when it becomes chronic, it can lead to long-term health challenges such as fatigue, joint pain, heart disease, and autoimmune disorders. Thankfully, what we eat has a profound impact on how our bodies respond to inflammation. By focusing on whole, nutrient-rich ingredients, you can support your body's natural ability to heal and thrive.

This cookbook offers 100 recipes that make anti-inflammatory eating simple and delicious. From energizing breakfasts to satisfying dinners and indulgent desserts, you'll discover meals that are easy to prepare, full of vibrant flavors, and packed with nutrients. Each recipe is crafted to help reduce inflammation, boost immunity, and make you feel your best—every single day.

You'll also find practical tips for meal prepping, batch cooking, and making ingredient swaps for seasonal produce or dietary needs. Whether you're just beginning your journey to healthier eating or looking for new inspiration, this book offers recipes and ideas that fit seamlessly into your daily life.

This isn't about restrictions or complicated rules; it's about celebrating balance, variety, and the joy of food. Cooking becomes an act of self-care and love, helping you feel connected to your health and the meals you create.

Let this cookbook inspire you to make everyday choices that support your health and happiness. These recipes are more than just meals—they're tools to empower and nurture you on the path to wellness. Your journey to a healthier, more vibrant life starts now, one delicious meal at a time.

Contents

Introduction 3

Breakfast/Brunch 8
Avocado Toast with Tomato and Hemp Seeds 9
Quinoa Salad with Spinach, Cherry Tomatoes, and Walnuts 10
Blueberry and Chia Overnight Oats 11
Smoked Salmon Bagel with Avocado 12
Sweet Potato and Apple Hash 13
Turmeric-Spiced Breakfast Scramble 14
Greek Yogurt with Honey and Walnuts 15
Veggie-Packed Frittata 16
Warm Quinoa Porridge with Berries 17
Almond Butter Banana Toast 18
Millet Porridge with Stewed Apples 19

Smoothies 20
Blueberry Spinach Power Smoothie 21
Berry and Almond Smoothie with Chia 22
Mango Ginger Green Smoothie 23
Cherry Beet Smoothie 24
Carrot and Orange Smoothie 25
Banana and Flaxseed Smoothie 26
Dragon Fruit and Kale Smoothie 27
Strawberry Mint Smoothie 28
Raspberry and Cocoa Smoothie 29

Lunches/Light Bites 30
Mediterranean Chickpea Salad with Olives 31
Spinach and Feta Stuffed Sweet Potatoes 32
Grilled Veggie Pita Pocket 33
Warm Lentil and Arugula Salad 34
Beet and Carrot Salad with Walnuts 35
Turmeric-Spiced Cauliflower Rice Bowl 36
Cucumber and Avocado Salad with Sesame 37
Sweet Potato and Black Bean Tacos 38
Grilled Portobello Mushroom Sandwich 39

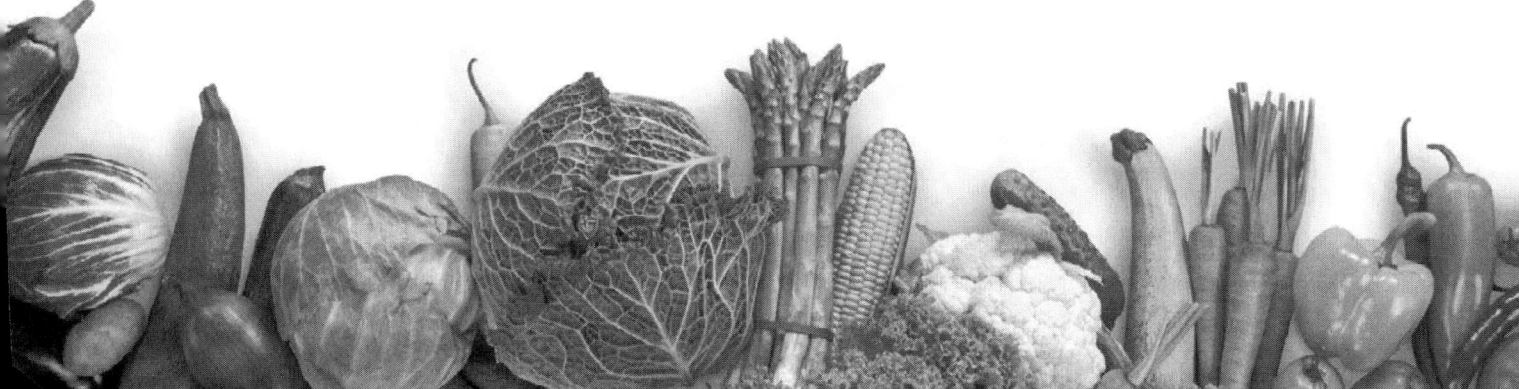

Dinners 40
Grilled Lemon Herb Chicken with Broccoli 41
Baked Salmon with Asparagus and Lemon 42
Turmeric-Coconut Chicken Curry 43
Shrimp and Zucchini Noodles with Garlic 44
Thai Basil Turkey Lettuce Wraps 45
Roasted Vegetable Stir-Fry with Tofu 46
Spinach and Chickpea Curry 47
Garlic and Herb Roasted Lamb with Carrots 48
Mediterranean Cod with Olive Tapenade 49

Budget-Friendly Recipes 50
Black Bean and Vegetable Soup 51
Chickpea and Tomato Stew 52
Simple Quinoa and Veggie Bowl 53
White Bean and Kale Soup 54
One-Pot Pasta with Veggies 55
Barley and Mushroom Risotto 56
Cauliflower and Lentil Curry 57
Whole Wheat Vegetable Stir-Fry 58
Sweet Potato and Black Bean Chili 59

Seasonal Produce Recipes 60
Spring Asparagus and Spinach Salad 61
Summer Tomato and Basil Gazpacho 62
Autumn Pumpkin and Lentil Stew 63
Summer Grilled Peach Salad 64
Spring Pea and Mint Soup 65
Summer Corn and Zucchini Sauté 66
Winter Beet and Orange Salad 67
Spring Radish and Avocado Bowl 68
Winter Carrot and Parsnip Roast 69

Superfoods Recipes 70
Quinoa Salad with Blueberries and Walnuts 71
Turmeric and Ginger Vegetable Soup 72
Chia Seed Pudding with Raspberries 73
Wild Salmon with Ginger and Sesame 74
Matcha Green Smoothie Bowl 75

Spinach and Sweet Potato Hash 76
Turmeric and Cauliflower Rice Bowl 77
Sweet Potato and Coconut Soup 78
Pumpkin Seed and Herb Pesto 79

Batch Cooking 80
Hearty Vegetable Soup 81
Black Bean Chili 82
Lentil and Vegetable Curry 83
Carrot and Ginger Soup 84
Vegetable and Barley Stew 85
Baked Chicken Thighs with Root Vegetables 86
Beef and Vegetable Stew 87
Mediterranean Eggplant Stew 88

Family-Friendly Meals 89
Turkey and Veggie Meatballs with Tomato Sauce 90
Chicken and Veggie Skewers 91
Fish Tacos with Mango Salsa 92
Sloppy Joes with Lentils 93
Mini Chicken and Avocado Tacos 94
Beef and Veggie Burgers 95
Shepherd's Pie with Lentils 96
Spaghetti Squash Marinara 97

Japanese & Mediterranean 98
Japanese Cucumber Salad 99
Mediterranean Baked Fish with Herbs 100
Miso Soup with Seaweed and Tofu 101
Japanese Eggplant Stir-Fry 102
Mediterranean Chickpea Stew 103
Mediterranean Farro Salad 104
Teriyaki Salmon with Steamed Veggies 105
Mediterranean Stuffed Peppers 106
Tofu and Vegetable Soba Noodles 107

30-Minute Meals 108
Lemon Garlic Shrimp with Asparagus 109
Turmeric-Spiced Chickpea and Pepper Stir-Fry 110
Quick Grilled Salmon with Quinoa 111

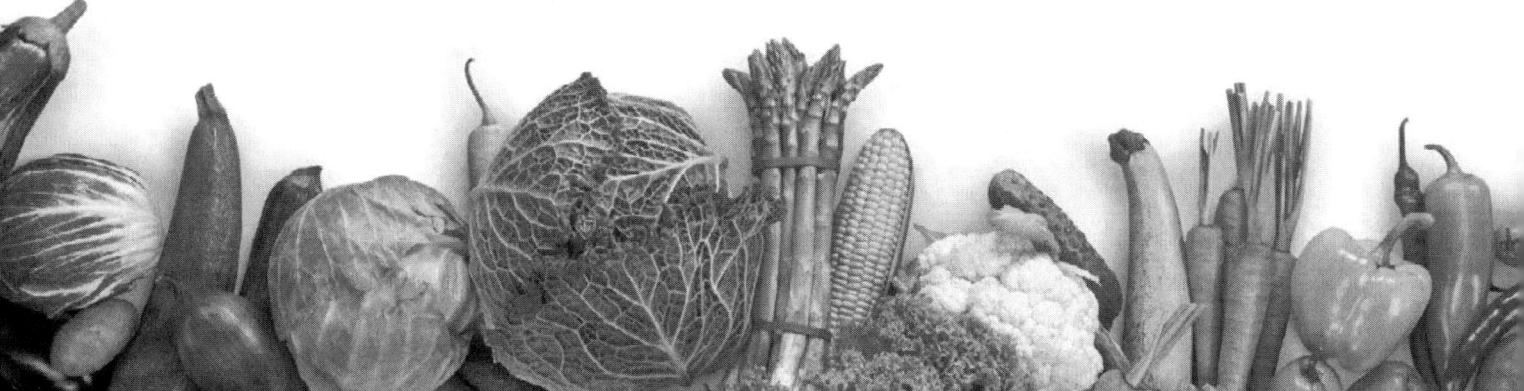

Balsamic Glazed Tofu with Zucchini.. 112
Garlic Lemon Chicken Thighs... 113
Quick Tuna and Avocado Salad.. 114
Easy Salmon and Spinach Salad... 115
Black Bean and Corn Tacos.. 116

One-Pot Dishes.. 117
One-Pot Lentil and Vegetable Stew... 118
One-Pot Turmeric Rice with Veggies.. 119
One-Pot Pasta with Fresh Herbs... 120
Sweet Potato and Black Bean Chili... 121
Thai Green Curry with Tofu.. 122
Wild Rice and Mushroom Soup.. 123
Mediterranean Chickpea Soup... 124
Indian-Spiced Lentil Stew... 125

Snacks: Sweet & Savory.. 126
Apple Slices with Almond Butter.. 127
Carrot Sticks with Hummus.. 128
Coconut and Almond Energy Balls... 129
Berry Chia Jam on Whole-Grain Crackers... 130
Baked Zucchini Chips.. 131
Sweet Potato Fries with Paprika... 132
Dark Chocolate and Walnut Clusters... 133
Apple and Cinnamon Bites... 134

Desserts 135
Dark Chocolate Avocado Mousse... 136
Coconut and Almond Energy Bars... 137
Lemon and Chia Seed Cookies.. 138
Baked Pears with Walnuts and Honey... 139
Matcha Green Tea Ice Cream... 140
Mango Coconut Sorbet... 141
Banana and Almond Butter Bites... 142
Pineapple and Ginger Popsicles.. 143

conclusion 144

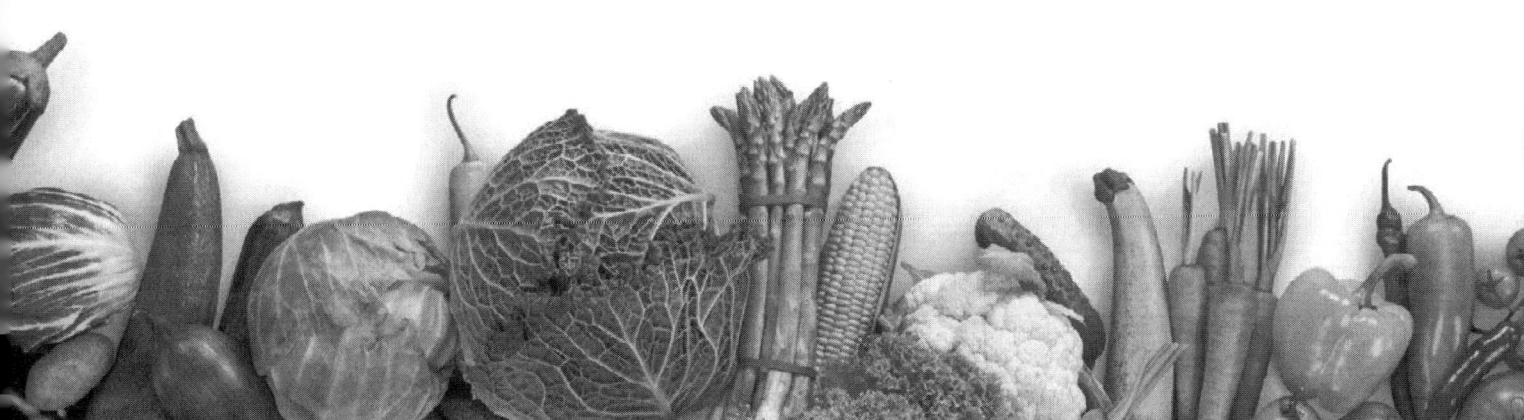

BREAKFAST/BRUNCH

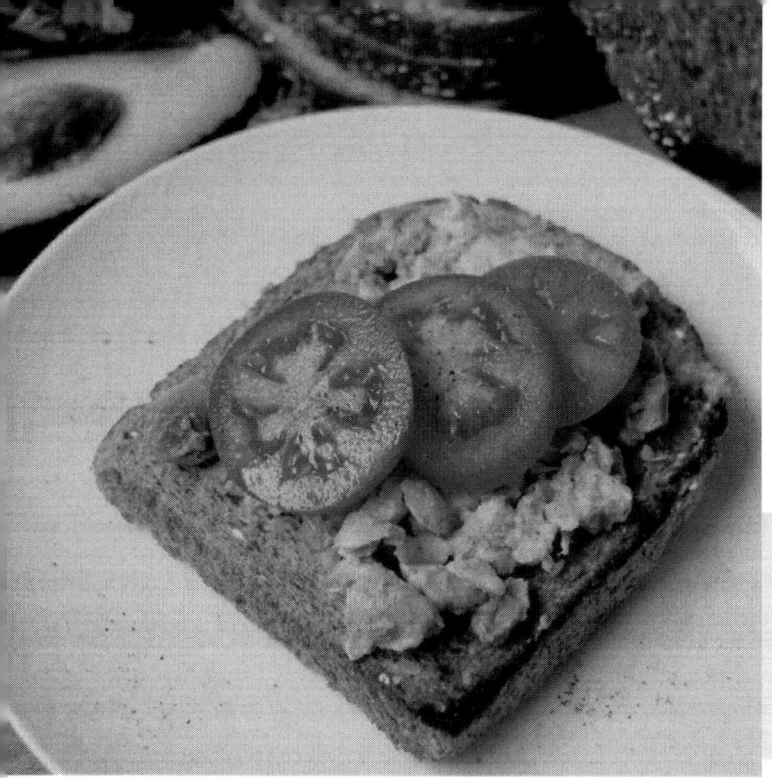

BREAKFAST/BRUNCH

AVOCADO TOAST WITH TOMATO AND HEMP SEEDS

Anti-Inflammatory Benefits:
Avocados are high in monounsaturated fats that help reduce inflammation, and tomatoes contain lycopene, an antioxidant known for its anti-inflammatory properties. Hemp seeds add omega-3 fatty acids, further supporting anti-inflammatory benefits.

PREP TIME: 5 MINS **COOK TIME:** 00 MINS **SERVING: 2** Portion Size: 1 toast per serving

INGREDIENTS

- 2 slices whole-grain bread (60 g total)
- 1 avocado (120 g), peeled and mashed
- 6 cherry tomatoes (60 g), sliced
- 2 tsp (10 g) hemp seeds
- Salt and pepper to taste
- Optional: red pepper flakes (just a pinch)

INSTRUCTIONS

1. Toast each slice of whole-grain bread until golden.
2. Smoothly spread mashed avocado on each slice of toast.
3. Top each with sliced cherry tomatoes and sprinkle with hemp seeds, salt, and pepper.
4. Sprinkle red pepper flakes if desired, then serve immediately.

EQUIPMENT NEEDED:
Knife, cutting board, and toaster or oven

 NUTRITIONAL INFORMATION (PER SERVING):

Calories: 210 kcal, Carbohydrates: 20 g, Protein: 5 g, Fat: 14 g, Fiber: 7 g

HEALTH BENEFITS:
Seasonal Produce Swap: Substitute cherry tomatoes with cucumber slices or radishes in the winter for a fresh, crisp alternative.
Dietary Substitutions: For a gluten-free option, use gluten-free bread.

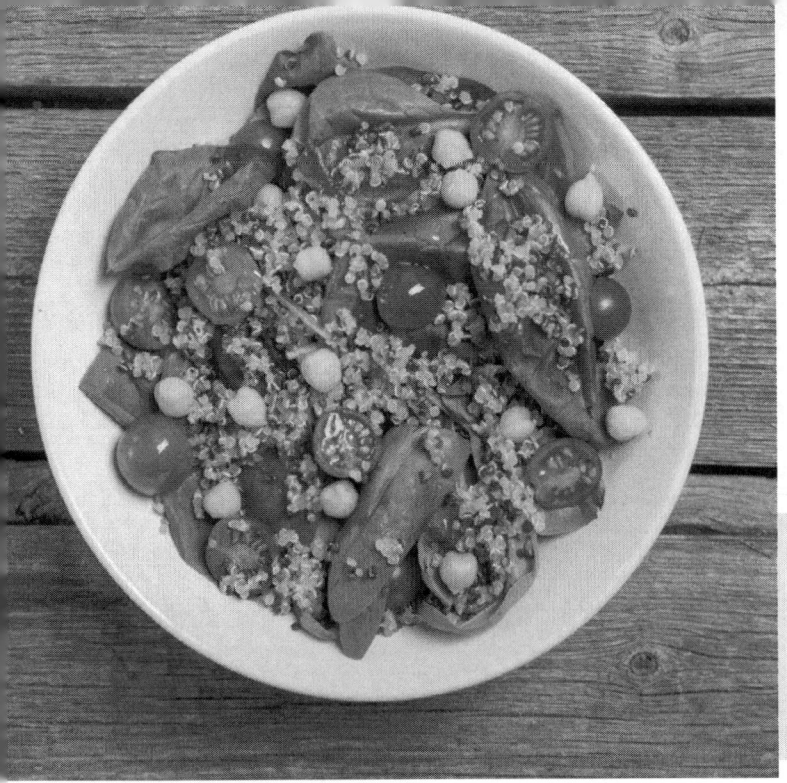

BREAKFAST/BRUNCH

QUINOA SALAD WITH SPINACH, CHERRY TOMATOES, AND WALNUTS

Anti-Inflammatory Benefits:
Quinoa is a complete protein and provides anti-inflammatory phytonutrients, spinach is packed with antioxidants, and walnuts offer omega-3 fatty acids, all of which help reduce inflammation in the body.

PREP TIME: 10 MINS   **COOK TIME:** 15 MINS   **SERVING:** 3 (1 bowl per serving)

INGREDIENTS

- 1/2 cup (90 g) quinoa, rinsed
- 1 1/2 cups (360 ml) water
- 3 cups (90 g) fresh spinach leaves
- 3/4 cup (120 g) cherry tomatoes, halved
- 3 tbsp (21 g) chopped walnuts
- 3 tbsp (45 ml) olive oil
- 1 1/2 tbsp (22.5 ml) balsamic vinegar
- Salt and pepper to taste

 EQUIPMENT NEEDED:
Saucepan, knife, cutting board, and mixing bowl

INSTRUCTIONS

1. In a saucepan, combine the quinoa and water. Get it to a boil, then decrease the stove heat, cover, and simmer for 15 minutes, or until the water is absorbed and the quinoa is tender. Remove from flame, then fluff with a fork.
2. In a large, deep-bottom bowl, combine the cooked quinoa, spinach leaves, cherry tomatoes, and walnuts.
3. Drizzle three tbsp oil and balsamic vinegar, then powder it with salt and crushed pepper.
4. Toss everything properly until well mixed, then serve immediately.

 NUTRITIONAL INFORMATION (PER SERVING):

Calories: 250 kcal, Carbohydrates: 22 g, Protein: 6 g, Fat: 16 g, Fiber: 5 g

HEALTH BENEFITS:
Seasonal Produce Swap: Substitute spinach with kale or arugula during the winter for a heartier texture.
Dietary Substitutions: For a nut-free option, replace walnuts with pumpkin seeds or sunflower seeds.

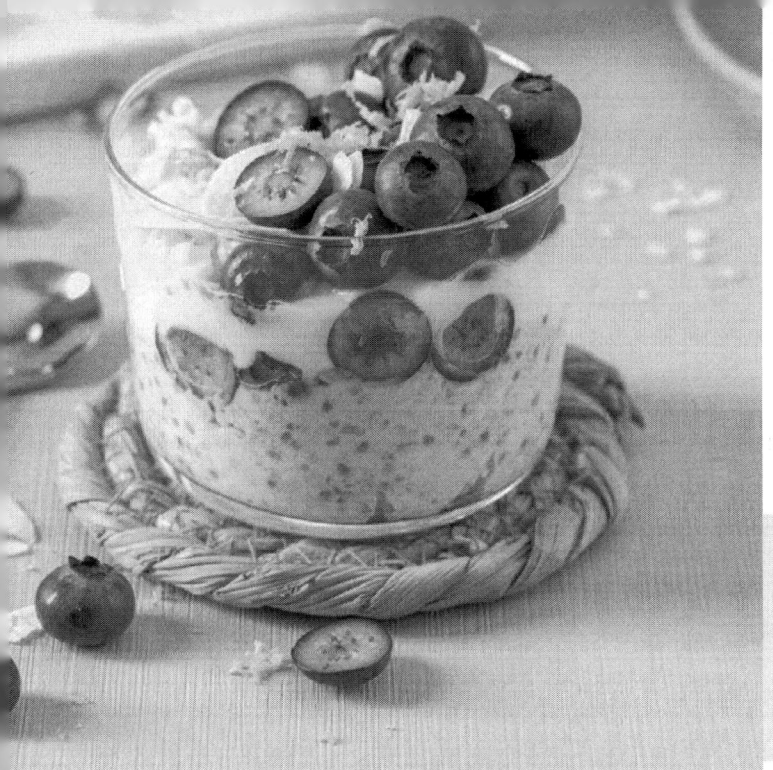

BREAKFAST/BRUNCH

BLUEBERRY AND CHIA OVERNIGHT OATS

Anti-Inflammatory Benefits:
Blueberries are rich in antioxidants, which help reduce inflammation and support overall health. Chia seeds provide omega-3 fatty acids, which also have anti-inflammatory properties.

PREP TIME: 5 MINS | **COOK TIME:** 00 MINS | **SERVING: 1** Portion Size: 1 bowl

INGREDIENTS

- 1/2 cup (40 g) rolled oats
- 1/2 cup (120 ml) almond milk
- 1 tbsp (15 g) chia seeds
- 1/4 cup (60 g) fresh blueberries
- 1/2 tsp (2.5 ml) vanilla extract (optional)
- 1 tsp (5 ml) honey or maple syrup (optional for sweetness)

INSTRUCTIONS

1. In a wide-mouth jar or bowl, combine the rolled oats, almond milk, chia seeds, and vanilla extract (if using).
2. Stir well to ensure the chia seeds are evenly distributed.
3. Cover and refrigerate for 4 hours (at least) or 6-8 hours.
4. In the morning, stir it a good bit and add fresh blueberries on top.
5. Drizzle sweetener (honey or maple syrup), if desired, before serving.

EQUIPMENT NEEDED:
Measuring cups and spoons, jar or bowl for soaking

NUTRITIONAL INFORMATION (PER SERVING):

Calories: 220 kcal, Carbohydrates: 34 g, Protein: 6 g, Fat: 7 g, Fiber: 8 g

HEALTH BENEFITS:
Seasonal Produce Swap: Substitute blueberries with seasonal fruits like strawberries, raspberries, or sliced apples in autumn.
Dietary Substitutions: For a nut-free option, use oat or coconut milk. For a lower-sugar option, skip the honey or maple syrup.

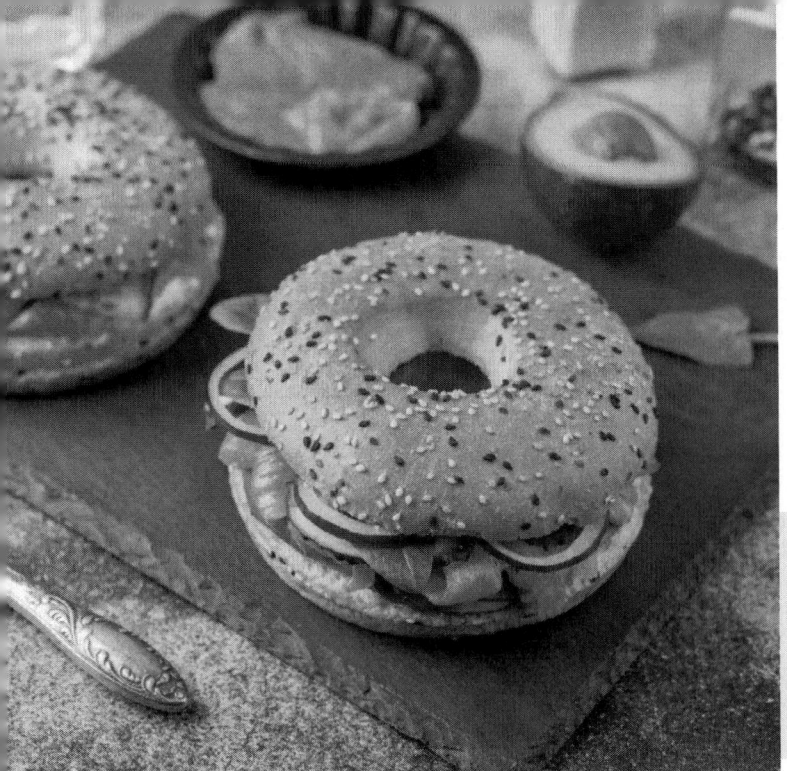

BREAKFAST/BRUNCH

SMOKED SALMON BAGEL WITH AVOCADO

Anti-Inflammatory Benefits:
Smoked salmon is rich in omega-3 fatty acids, which help reduce inflammation, while avocado provides healthy fats and fiber for heart health.

PREP TIME: 5 MINS   **COOK TIME:** 00 MINS   **SERVING: 1** 1 bagel per serving

INGREDIENTS

- 2 whole-grain bagels, halved and toasted
- 100 g smoked salmon
- 1/2 avocado (75 g), sliced
- 1/4 cup (30 g) cream cheese
- 1 tsp (5 ml) lemon juice
- Fresh dill or chives for garnish (optional)

INSTRUCTIONS

1. Spread cream cheese evenly on each toasted bagel half.
2. Layer with smoked salmon slices and avocado.
3. Drizzle with lemon juice and garnish with dill or chives, if desired.
4. Serve immediately for a quick, satisfying breakfast or brunch.

 EQUIPMENT NEEDED:
Knife, toaster

 NUTRITIONAL INFORMATION (PER SERVING):

Calories: 300 kcal, Carbohydrates: 32 g, Protein: 15 g, Fat: 12 g, Fiber: 4 g

HEALTH BENEFITS:
Seasonal Produce Swap: Add sliced cucumber or radishes for a refreshing crunch.
Dietary Substitutions: Use dairy-free cream cheese for a vegan alternative.

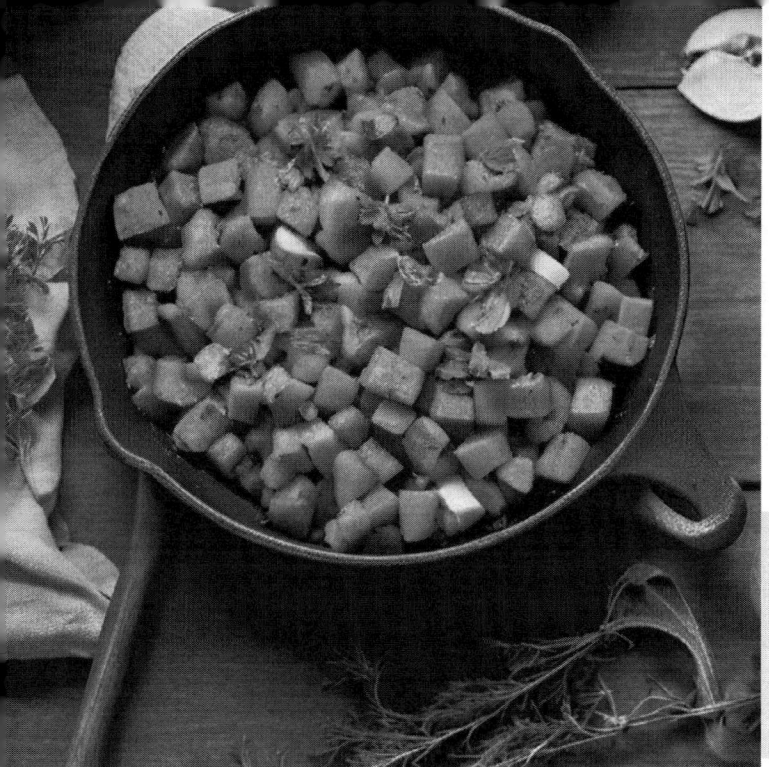

BREAKFAST/BRUNCH

SWEET POTATO AND APPLE HASH

Anti-Inflammatory Benefits:
Sweet potatoes are high in beta-carotene and fiber, which keep up the immune function and reduce inflammation. Apples are rich in antioxidants and fiber, aiding digestion and combating inflammation

PREP TIME:
10 MINS

COOK TIME:
15 MINS

SERVING: 2
Portion Size: 1 bowl per serving

INGREDIENTS

- 1 medium sweet potato (150 g), peeled and diced
- 1 apple (100 g), cored and diced
- 1/2 red onion (50 g), diced
- 1/2 bell pepper (50 g), diced
- 1/2 tsp (1 g) ground cinnamon
- Salt and pepper to taste
- Fresh parsley, chopped (for garnish, optional)

EQUIPMENT NEEDED:
Knife, cutting board, skillet or frying pan, spatula

INSTRUCTIONS

1. In a skillet over moderate stove flame, add a small amount of oil and add sweet potato. Sauté for about 8–10 minutes until it begins to soften.
2. Add apple, red onion, and bell pepper to the skillet. Stir and cook for more 5–7 minutes, until everything is tender and slightly caramelized.
3. Sprinkle with cinnamon, salt, and pepper, and stir well.
4. Spread fresh parsley on top, then serve warm.

 NUTRITIONAL INFORMATION (PER SERVING):

Calories: 180 kcal, Carbohydrates: 35 g, Protein: 2 g, Fat: 4 g, Fiber: 6 g

HEALTH BENEFITS:
Seasonal Produce Swap: Swap the apple for pear or add butternut squash in place of sweet potato in autumn.
Dietary Substitutions: For added protein, add a handful of cooked chickpeas during the last few minutes of cooking.

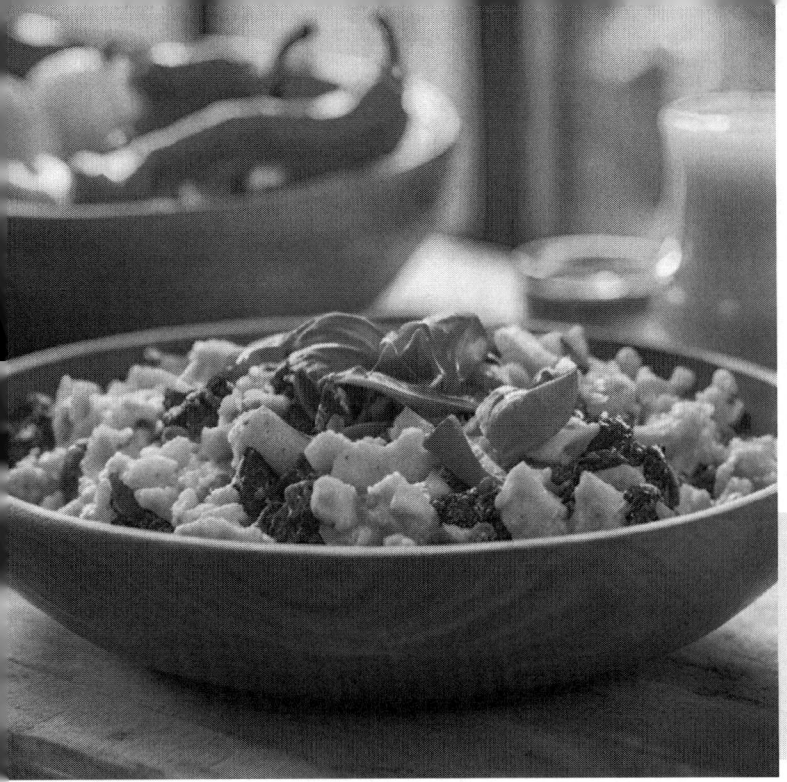

BREAKFAST/BRUNCH

TURMERIC-SPICED BREAKFAST SCRAMBLE

Anti-Inflammatory Benefits:
Turmeric contains curcumin, a powerful anti-inflammatory compound, while bell peppers add vitamin C and antioxidants to further support immune health.

PREP TIME: 5 MINS **COOK TIME:** 10 MINS **SERVING: 2** Portion Size: 1 plate per serving

INGREDIENTS

- 4 large eggs
- 1/2 tsp (1 g) ground turmeric
- 1/4 cup (60 ml) almond milk
- 1/2 red bell pepper (50 g), diced
- 1/2 cup (30 g) fresh spinach, chopped
- Salt and pepper to taste
- Fresh parsley or chives for garnish (optional)

INSTRUCTIONS

1. Take a large, deep-bottom bowl and whisk the eggs, turmeric, almond milk, salt, and pepper until well combined.
2. In a skillet over moderate stove flame, add a small amount of oil and add bell pepper. Sauté for 2–3 minutes until it starts to soften.
3. Add spinach, then pour in the egg mixture.
4. Cook, stirring softly, until the eggs are set and fluffy, about 5 minutes.
5. Spread fresh parsley or chives on top, then serve warm.

 NUTRITIONAL INFORMATION (PER SERVING):

Calories: 140 kcal, Carbohydrates: 4 g, Protein: 10 g, Fat: 10 g, Fiber: 1 g

HEALTH BENEFITS:
Seasonal Produce Swap: Substitute bell pepper with zucchini or mushrooms, or use kale in place of spinach.
Dietary Substitutions: For a dairy-free option, use any plant-based milk as listed.

EQUIPMENT NEEDED:
Mixing bowl, skillet or frying pan, spatula

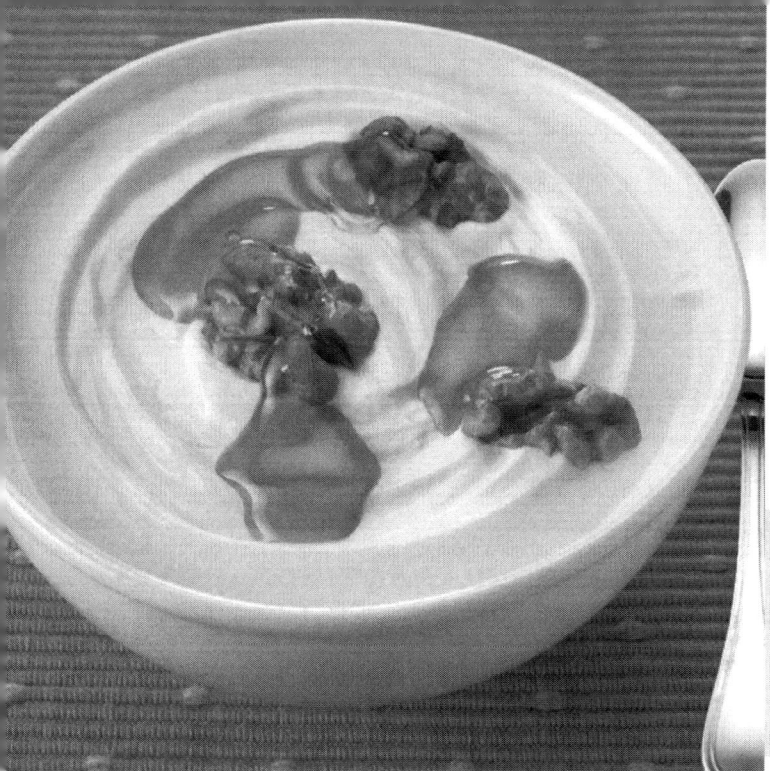

BREAKFAST/BRUNCH

GREEK YOGURT WITH HONEY AND WALNUTS

Anti-Inflammatory Benefits:
Greek yogurt provides probiotics that support gut health and reduce inflammation, while walnuts are rich in omega-3 fatty acids, which also help to reduce inflammation.

PREP TIME: 5 MINS   **COOK TIME:** 00 MINS   **SERVING:** 1 Portion Size: : 1 bowl

INGREDIENTS

- 1 cup (240 g) Greek yogurt (plain, unsweetened)
- 1 tbsp (15 ml) honey
- 2 tbsp (15 g) walnuts, chopped

INSTRUCTIONS

1. Take a deep-bottom bowl, add Greek yogurt, and drizzle honey on top.
2. Sprinkle with chopped walnuts and serve immediately.

 EQUIPMENT NEEDED:
Spoon, small bowl

 NUTRITIONAL INFORMATION (PER SERVING):

Calories: 220 kcal, Carbohydrates: 19 g, Protein: 14 g, Fat: 10 g, Fiber: 1 g

HEALTH BENEFITS:
Seasonal Produce Swap: SAdd fresh berries or pomegranate seeds when in season.
Dietary Substitutions: Use almond yogurt as a dairy-free option, and substitute honey with a small amount of maple syrup if desired.

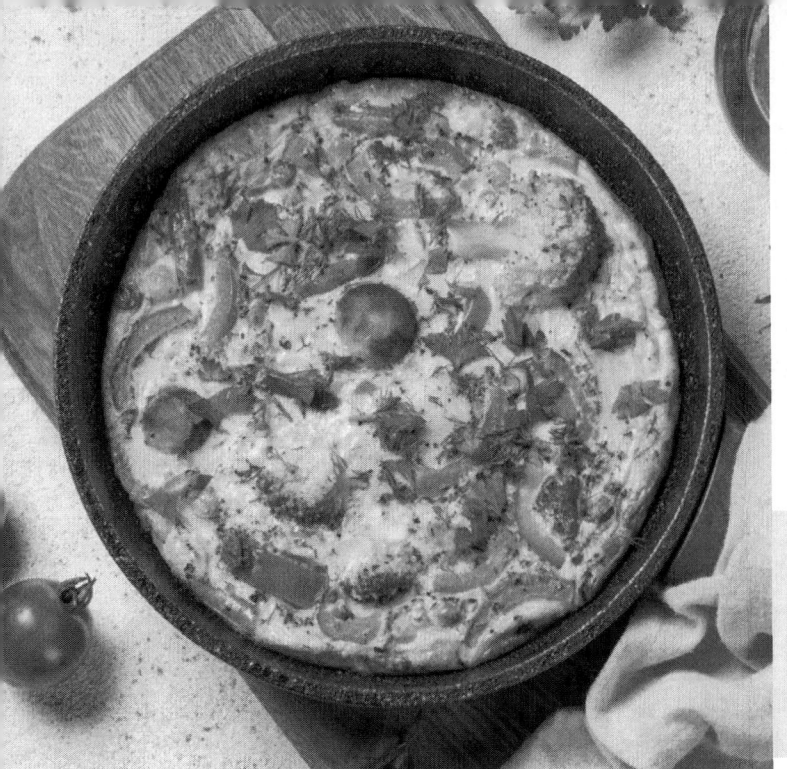

BREAKFAST/BRUNCH

VEGGIE-PACKED FRITTATA

Anti-Inflammatory Benefits:
This frittata is loaded with vegetables rich in antioxidants and vitamins that keep up the immune health and reduce inflammation.

PREP TIME: 10 MINS | **COOK TIME:** 20 MINS | **SERVING: 3** Portion Size: 1 slice per serving

INGREDIENTS

- 6 large eggs
- 1/4 cup (60 ml) almond milk
- 1/2 red bell pepper (50 g), diced
- 1/2 zucchini (50 g), diced
- 1/2 cup (30 g) fresh spinach, chopped
- 1/4 cup (30 g) cherry tomatoes, halved
- Salt and pepper to taste
- Fresh basil or parsley for garnish (optional)

EQUIPMENT NEEDED:
Knife, cutting board, skillet or oven-safe pan, mixing bowl, spatula

INSTRUCTIONS

1. Preheat oven to 350°F (175°C).
2. Take a large, deep-bottom bowl and toss the eggs with almond milk, salt, and pepper until well combined.
3. In an oven-safe skillet over moderate stove flame, add a small amount of oil and sauté the bell pepper and zucchini for 3–4 minutes until softened.
4. Add spinach and cherry tomato slices and cook for another 2 minutes.
5. Ladle egg mixture over the veggies and cook for 2–3 minutes.
6. Transfer the skillet and bake for 10–12 minutes until the frittata is set in the center.
7. Spread fresh basil or parsley on top and serve warm.

 NUTRITIONAL INFORMATION (PER SERVING):

Calories: 140 kcal, Carbohydrates: 5 g, Protein: 10 g, Fat: 9 g, Fiber: 2 g

HEALTH BENEFITS:
Seasonal Produce Swap: Substitute spinach with kale or add mushrooms and onions for variety.
Dietary Substitutions: For a dairy-free option, use any plant-based milk as listed.

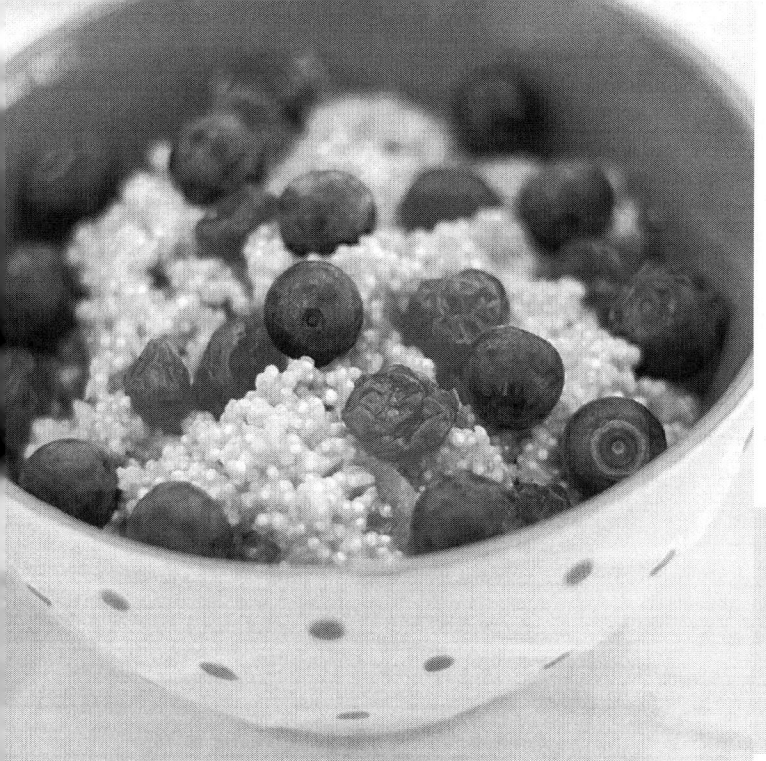

WARM QUINOA PORRIDGE WITH BERRIES

BREAKFAST/BRUNCH

Anti-Inflammatory Benefits:
Quinoa is a complete protein and provides essential amino acids and fiber, while berries are high in antioxidants that reduce inflammation.

PREP TIME: 5 MINS | **COOK TIME:** 15 MINS | **SERVING: 2** Portion Size: : 1 bowl per serving

INGREDIENTS

- 1/2 cup (90 g) quinoa, rinsed
- 1 cup (240 ml) almond milk
- 1/4 tsp (1 g) ground cinnamon
- 1/2 cup (75 g) mixed berries (blueberries, raspberries, strawberries)
- 1 tsp (5 ml) honey or maple syrup (optional for sweetness)

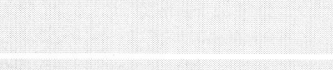 **EQUIPMENT NEEDED:**
Saucepan, spoon, bowl

INSTRUCTIONS

1. In a saucepan, throw in quinoa, almond milk, and cinnamon. Get it to a boil, then decrease the stove heat and simmer for 15 minutes, stirring occasionally, until the quinoa gets a tender texture and most of the liquid is absorbed.
2. Divide the prepared quinoa into two wide-mouth bowls and top with mixed berries.
3. Drizzle sweetener (honey or maple syrup) if desired and serve warm.

 NUTRITIONAL INFORMATION (PER SERVING):

Calories: 190 kcal, Carbohydrates: 30 g, Protein: 6 g, Fat: 5 g, Fiber: 5 g

HEALTH BENEFITS:
Seasonal Produce Swap: Use sliced apples or pears in the fall or pomegranate seeds in winter.
Dietary Substitutions: For a lower-sugar option, omit the honey or maple syrup.

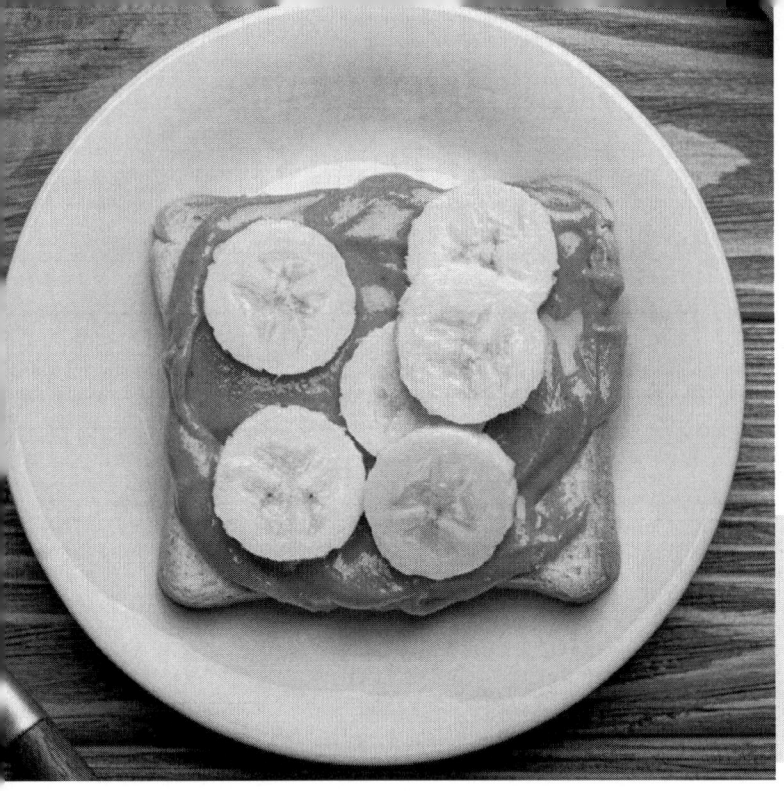

BREAKFAST/BRUNCH

ALMOND BUTTER BANANA TOAST

Anti-Inflammatory Benefits:
Almond butter provides healthy fats and vitamin E, which support skin and immune health. Bananas offer potassium and fiber to support digestion and reduce inflammation.

 PREP TIME: 5 MINS

 **COOK TIME:** 00 MINS

 **SERVING: 1** Portion Size: 1 toast

INGREDIENTS

- 1 slice whole-grain bread (30 g)
- 1 tbsp (15 g) almond butter
- 1/2 banana (50 g), sliced
- Optional toppings: chia seeds or a sprinkle of cinnamon

INSTRUCTIONS

1. Toast the slice of whole-grain bread until golden.
2. Spread almond butter evenly over the toast.
3. Top with banana slices and add optional toppings if desired, then serve immediately.

EQUIPMENT NEEDED:
Knife, toaster or oven

 NUTRITIONAL INFORMATION (PER SERVING):

Calories: 200 kcal, Carbohydrates: 25 g, Protein: 5 g, Fat: 10 g, Fiber: 4 g

HEALTH BENEFITS:
Seasonal Produce Swap: Substitute banana with fresh apple slices or pear slices in the fall.
Dietary Substitutions: For a nut-free option, use sunflower seed butter.

18

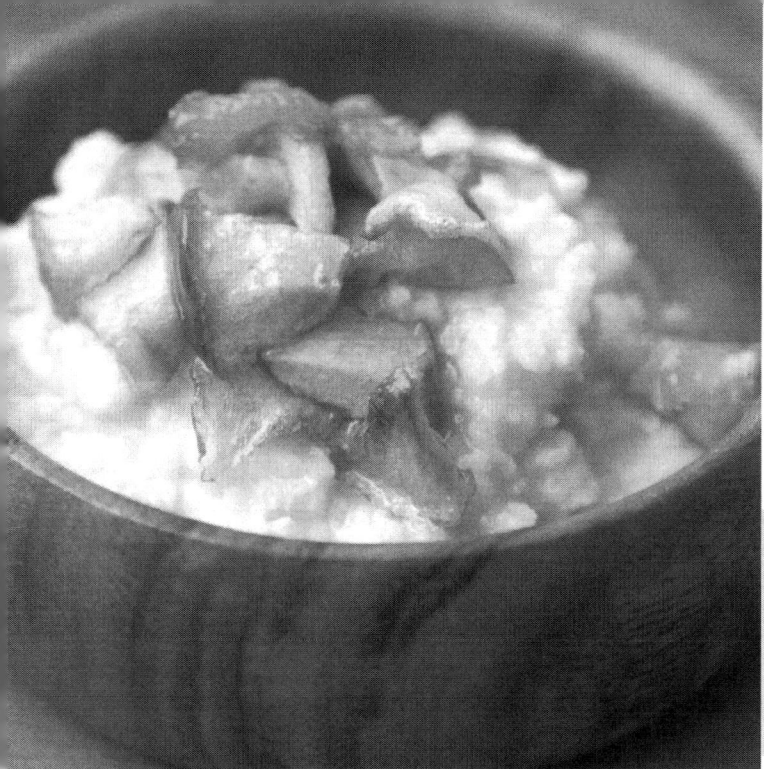

BREAKFAST/BRUNCH

MILLET PORRIDGE WITH STEWED APPLES

Anti-Inflammatory Benefits:
Millet is a gluten-free grain high in fiber, which supports digestion. Apples contain antioxidants and fiber that help combat inflammation.

PREP TIME: 10 MINS **COOK TIME:** 20 MINS **SERVING: 2** Portion Size: : 1 bowl per serving

INGREDIENTS

- 1/2 cup (90 g) millet, rinsed
- 1 1/2 cups (360 ml) water
- 1/2 cup (120 ml) almond milk
- 1 apple (100 g), diced
- 1/2 tsp (1 g) ground cinnamon
- 1 tsp (5 ml) honey or maple syrup (optional)

INSTRUCTIONS

1. In a saucepan, combine the millet and water. Get it to a boil, then decrease the stove heat and simmer for 15 minutes until the millet is tender and most of the water is absorbed.
2. While cooking, use the other small saucepan, add diced apple, cinnamon, and a splash of water. Cook over low flame for 5 minutes until the apples are softened and fragrant.
3. Once the millet is cooked, Toss in the almond milk and cook for another 2–3 minutes until creamy.
4. Divide the millet porridge into two bowls, top with the stewed apples, and drizzle with honey or maple syrup if desired.

EQUIPMENT NEEDED:
Saucepan, spoon, bowl

NUTRITIONAL INFORMATION (PER SERVING):

Calories: 220 kcal, Carbohydrates: 38 g, Protein: 5 g, Fat: 4 g, Fiber: 5 g

HEALTH BENEFITS:

Seasonal Produce Swap: Substitute apples with pears in autumn or fresh berries in the summer.
Dietary Substitutions: For a lower-sugar option, omit the honey or maple syrup.

SMOOTHIES

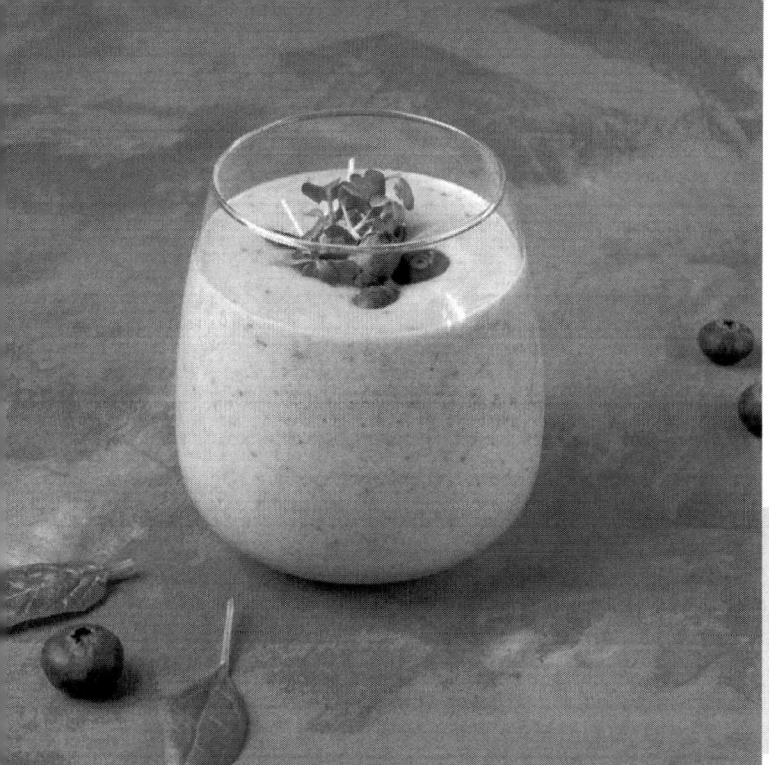

SMOOTHIES

BLUEBERRY SPINACH POWER SMOOTHIE

Anti-Inflammatory Benefits:
Blueberries are packed with antioxidants that help reduce inflammation, while spinach provides a dose of anti-inflammatory vitamins and minerals like magnesium and vitamin E.

PREP TIME: 5 MINS **COOK TIME:** 00 MINS **SERVING: 1** Portion Size: : 1 glass

INGREDIENTS

- 1/2 cup (75 g) fresh blueberries
- 1 cup (30 g) fresh spinach leaves
- 1/2 banana (50 g), sliced
- 1/2 cup (120 ml) almond milk
- 1 tsp (5 ml) honey or maple syrup (optional for sweetness)

INSTRUCTIONS

1. Combine all ingredients in a blender.
2. Blend on full power until the ingredient's texture looks smooth and creamy. Add more almond milk for the wished consistency.
3. Pour into a glass and serve immediately.

 EQUIPMENT NEEDED:

Blender, measuring cups

 **NUTRITIONAL INFORMATION** (PER SERVING):

Calories: 130 kcal, Carbohydrates: 25 g, Protein: 3 g, Fat: 2 g, Fiber: 4 g

HEALTH BENEFITS:

Seasonal Produce Swap: Substitute blueberries with strawberries or blackberries when in season.
Dietary Substitutions: For a nut-free option, use oat milk instead of almond milk.

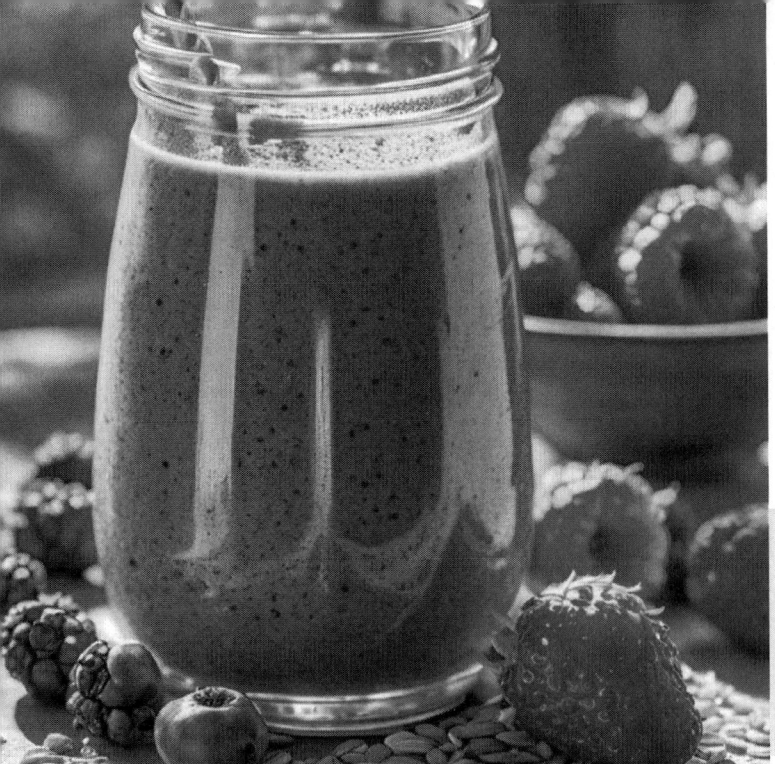

SMOOTHIES

BERRY AND ALMOND SMOOTHIE WITH CHIA

Anti-Inflammatory Benefits:
Mixed berries provide antioxidants, while chia seeds deliver omega-3 fatty acids, both of which help combat inflammation.

PREP TIME:
5 MINS

COOK TIME:
00 MINS

SERVING: 1
Portion Size: 1 glass

INGREDIENTS

- 1/2 cup (75 g) mixed berries (blueberries, raspberries, strawberries)
- 1 cup (240 ml) almond milk
- 1 tbsp (15 g) almond butter
- 1 tsp (5 g) chia seeds

EQUIPMENT NEEDED:
Blender, measuring cups

INSTRUCTIONS

1. Combine all ingredients in a blender.
2. Blend on full power until the ingredient's texture looks smooth and creamy. Adjust with almond milk for the desired consistency.
3. Pour into a glass and serve immediately.

NUTRITIONAL INFORMATION (PER SERVING):

Calories: 180 kcal, Carbohydrates: 20 g, Protein: 5 g, Fat: 9 g, Fiber: 6 g

HEALTH BENEFITS:
Seasonal Produce Swap: Use frozen berries in winter or fresh seasonal berries in spring and summer.
Dietary Substitutions: Replace almond butter with sunflower seed butter for a nut-free option.

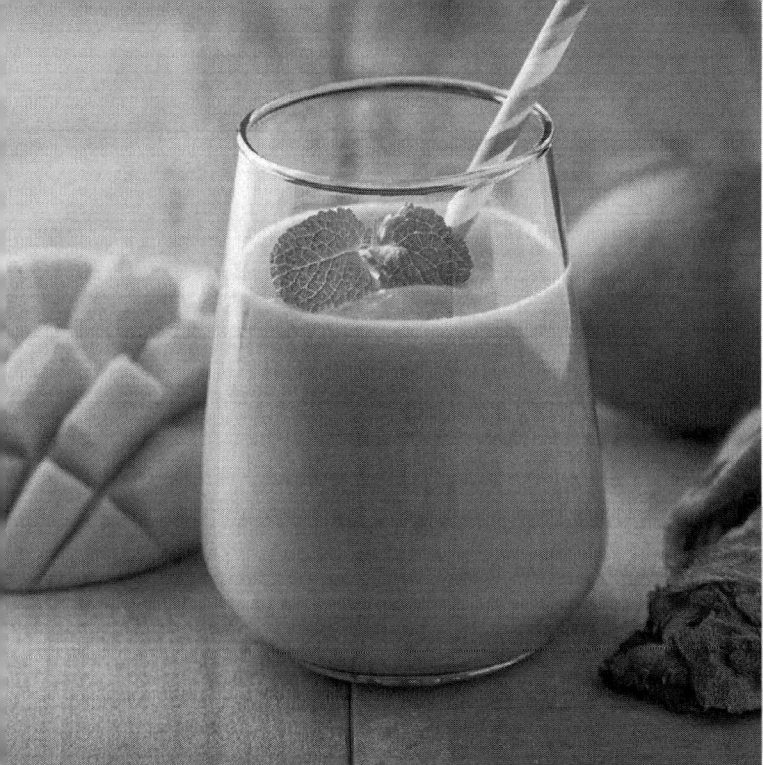

MANGO GINGER GREEN SMOOTHIE

SMOOTHIES

Anti-Inflammatory Benefits:
Mango is rich in vitamins A and C, which have anti-inflammatory properties. Ginger is a well-known anti-inflammatory spice that helps reduce inflammation and support digestion.

PREP TIME: 5 MINS | **COOK TIME:** 00 MINS | **SERVING: 1** Portion Size: : 1 glass

INGREDIENTS

- 1/2 cup (75 g) fresh mango chunks
- 1 cup (30 g) fresh spinach leaves
- 1/2 tsp (1 g) freshly grated ginger
- 1/2 cup (120 ml) coconut water
- 1 tsp (5 ml) honey or maple syrup (optional)

 EQUIPMENT NEEDED:
Blender, measuring cups

INSTRUCTIONS

1. Combine all ingredients in a blender.
2. Blend on full power until the ingredient's texture looks smooth and creamy. Adjust with coconut water for desired consistency.
3. Pour into a glass and serve immediately.

 NUTRITIONAL INFORMATION (PER SERVING):

Calories: 120 kcal, Carbohydrates: 24 g, Protein: 2 g, Fat: 1 g, Fiber: 3 g

HEALTH BENEFITS:
Seasonal Produce Swap: Use pineapple chunks instead of mango for variety.
Dietary Substitutions: Skip the honey for a lower-sugar option.

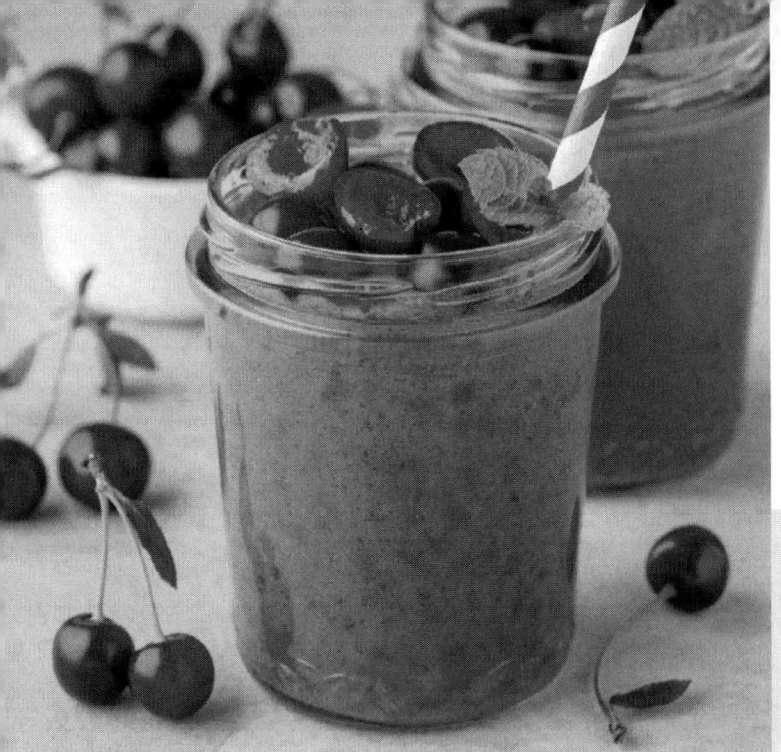

CHERRY BEET SMOOTHIE

SMOOTHIES

Anti-Inflammatory Benefits:
Beets are a natural source of nitrates, which reduce inflammation, while cherries are rich in antioxidants and anti-inflammatory compounds.

PREP TIME: 5 MINS   **COOK TIME:** 00 MINS   **SERVING:** 1 Portion Size: 1 glass

INGREDIENTS

- 1/2 cup (75 g) fresh cherries, pitted
- 1/4 cup (50 g) cooked beetroot, diced
- 1/2 banana (50 g), sliced
- 1/2 cup (120 ml) almond milk

INSTRUCTIONS

1. Combine all ingredients in a blender.
2. Blend on full power until the ingredient's texture looks smooth and creamy. Adjust with almond milk for the desired consistency.
3. Pour into a glass and serve immediately.

 EQUIPMENT NEEDED:
Blender, measuring cups

 NUTRITIONAL INFORMATION (PER SERVING):

Calories: 140 kcal, Carbohydrates: 30 g, Protein: 3 g, Fat: 1 g, Fiber: 4 g

HEALTH BENEFITS:
Seasonal Produce Swap: Use frozen cherries in winter if fresh ones are unavailable.
Dietary Substitutions: Replace almond milk with oat or rice milk for a nut-free option.

24

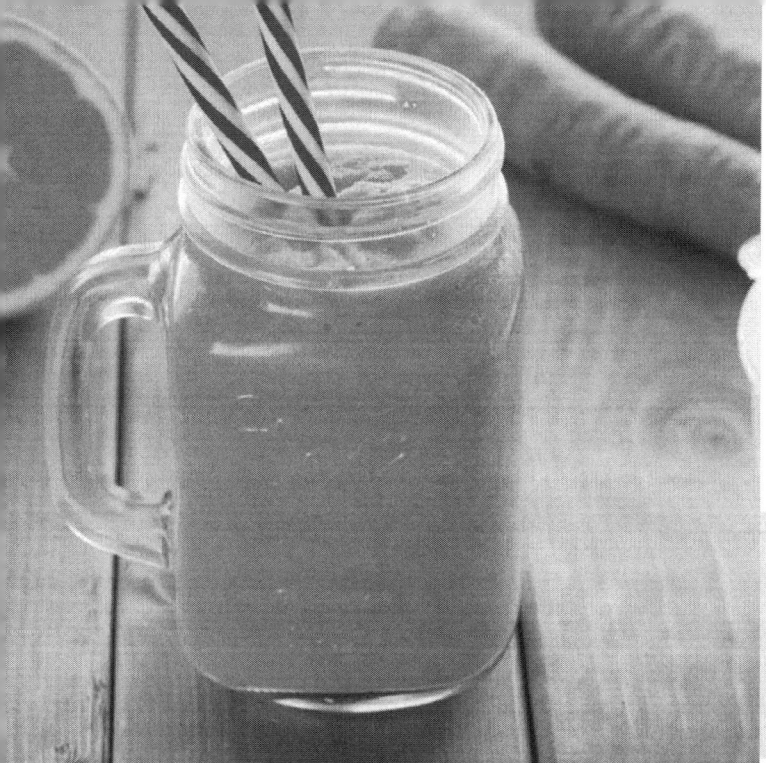

SMOOTHIES

CARROT AND ORANGE SMOOTHIE

Anti-Inflammatory Benefits:
Carrots are high in beta-carotene, a powerful antioxidant, while oranges provide vitamin C to help reduce inflammation and support immunity.

PREP TIME: 5 MINS | **COOK TIME:** 00 MINS | **SERVING: 1** Portion Size: : 1 glass

INGREDIENTS

- 1 medium carrot (50 g), peeled and diced
- 1/2 orange (75 g), peeled and segmented
- 1/2 cup (120 ml) coconut water
- 1/4 tsp (1 g) freshly grated ginger

INSTRUCTIONS

1. Combine all ingredients in a blender.
2. Blend on full power until the ingredient's texture looks smooth. Add more coconut water for the right consistency.
3. Pour into a glass and serve immediately.

 EQUIPMENT NEEDED:
Blender, measuring cups

 NUTRITIONAL INFORMATION (PER SERVING):

Calories: 90 kcal, Carbohydrates: 20 g, Protein: 1 g, Fat: 0 g, Fiber: 3 g

HEALTH BENEFITS:
Seasonal Produce Swap: Add a small apple for extra sweetness in autumn.
Dietary Substitutions: Replace coconut water with almond milk for a creamier texture.

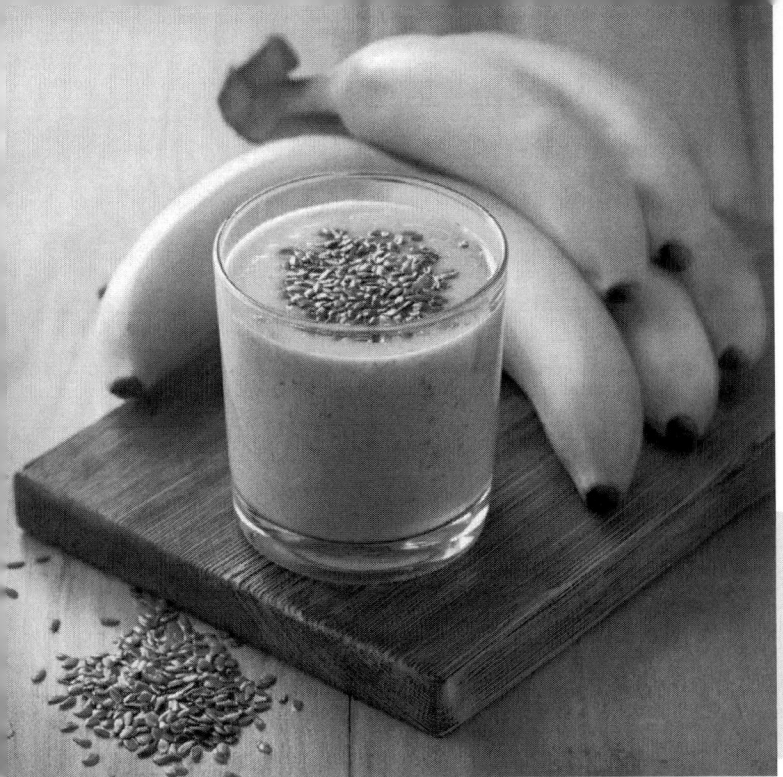

SMOOTHIES

BANANA AND FLAXSEED SMOOTHIE

Anti-Inflammatory Benefits:
Bananas are rich in potassium and fiber, supporting heart health and digestion, while flaxseeds are an excellent source of omega-3 fatty acids and lignans, which reduce inflammation.

PREP TIME: 5 MINS | **COOK TIME:** 00 MINS | **SERVING:** 1 Portion Size: 1 glass

INGREDIENTS

- 1 ripe banana (100 g), sliced
- 1 cup (240 ml) almond milk
- 1 tsp (5 g) ground flaxseed
- 1/2 tsp (2.5 ml) vanilla extract (optional)

INSTRUCTIONS

1. Combine all ingredients in a blender.
2. Blend on full power until the ingredient's texture looks smooth and creamy. Adjust with almond milk for the desired consistency.
3. Pour into a glass and serve immediately.

EQUIPMENT NEEDED:
Blender, measuring cups

 NUTRITIONAL INFORMATION (PER SERVING):

Calories: 150 kcal, Carbohydrates: 30 g, Protein: 3 g, Fat: 3 g, Fiber: 4 g

HEALTH BENEFITS:
Seasonal Produce Swap: Add frozen mango or pineapple chunks for a tropical twist.
Dietary Substitutions: Use oat or rice milk for a nut-free option.

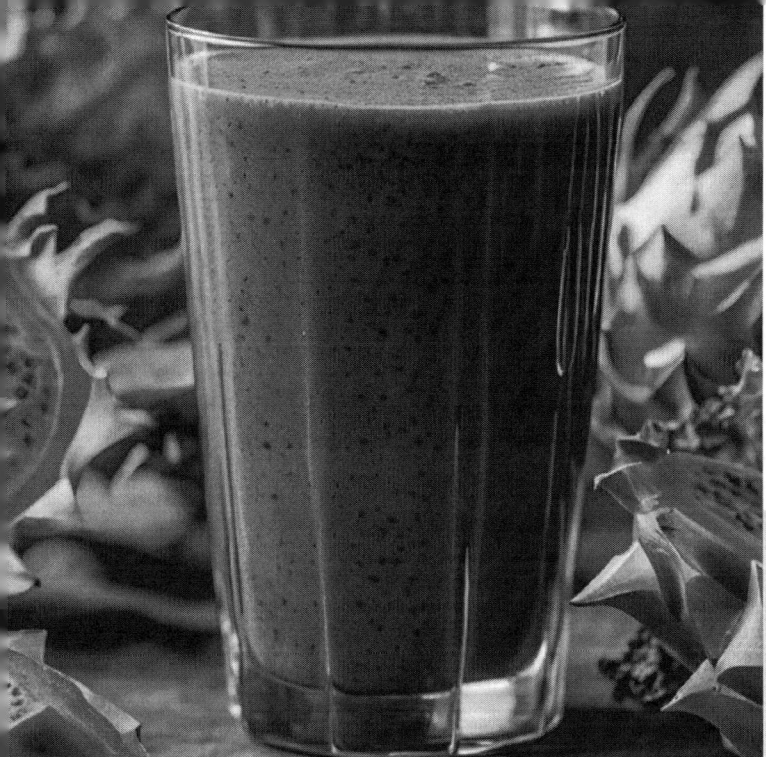

SMOOTHIES

DRAGON FRUIT AND KALE SMOOTHIE

Anti-Inflammatory Benefits:
Dragon fruit is rich in antioxidants like vitamin C, while kale is packed with anti-inflammatory compounds like quercetin and kaempferol, making this smoothie a nutrient powerhouse.

PREP TIME: 5 MINS   **COOK TIME:** 00 MINS   **SERVING: 1** Portion Size: : 1 glass

INGREDIENTS

- 1/2 cup (100 g) dragon fruit (fresh or frozen), diced
- 1 cup (30 g) fresh kale leaves, chopped
- 1/2 cup (120 ml) coconut water
- 1/2 banana (50 g), sliced

 EQUIPMENT NEEDED:
Blender, measuring cups

INSTRUCTIONS

1. Combine all ingredients in a blender.
2. Blend on full power until the ingredient's texture looks smooth and creamy. Add more coconut water if needed for the desired consistency.
3. Pour into a glass and serve immediately.

 **NUTRITIONAL INFORMATION** (PER SERVING):

Calories: 110 kcal, Carbohydrates: 25 g, Protein: 2 g, Fat: 0 g, Fiber: 4 g

HEALTH BENEFITS:
Seasonal Produce Swap: ASubstitute dragon fruit with mango or peach when dragon fruit is unavailable.
Dietary Substitutions: Replace coconut water with almond milk for a creamier texture.

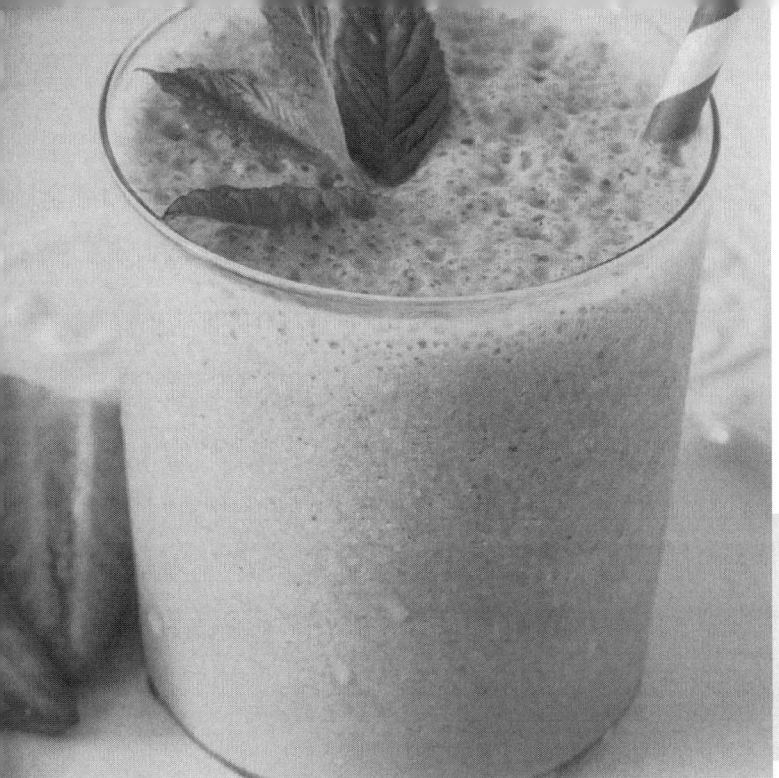

SMOOTHIES

STRAWBERRY MINT SMOOTHIE

Anti-Inflammatory Benefits:
Strawberries are loaded with antioxidants and vitamin C, while fresh mint helps soothe the digestive system and reduce inflammation.

PREP TIME:
5 MINS

COOK TIME:
00 MINS

SERVING: 1
Portion Size: 1 glass

INGREDIENTS

- 1/2 cup (75 g) fresh strawberries
- 1/2 cup (120 ml) almond milk
- 5–6 fresh mint leaves
- 1 tsp (5 ml) honey or maple syrup (optional for sweetness)

INSTRUCTIONS

1. Combine all ingredients in a blender.
2. Blend on full power until the ingredient's texture looks smooth and creamy. Add more almond milk for the desired consistency.
3. Pour into a glass and serve immediately.

EQUIPMENT NEEDED:
Blender, measuring cups

NUTRITIONAL INFORMATION (PER SERVING):

Calories: 90 kcal, Carbohydrates: 18 g, Protein: 2 g, Fat: 2 g, Fiber: 3 g

HEALTH BENEFITS:
Seasonal Produce Swap: Use raspberries or blueberries as a substitute for strawberries.
Dietary Substitutions: Skip the honey for a lower-sugar option.

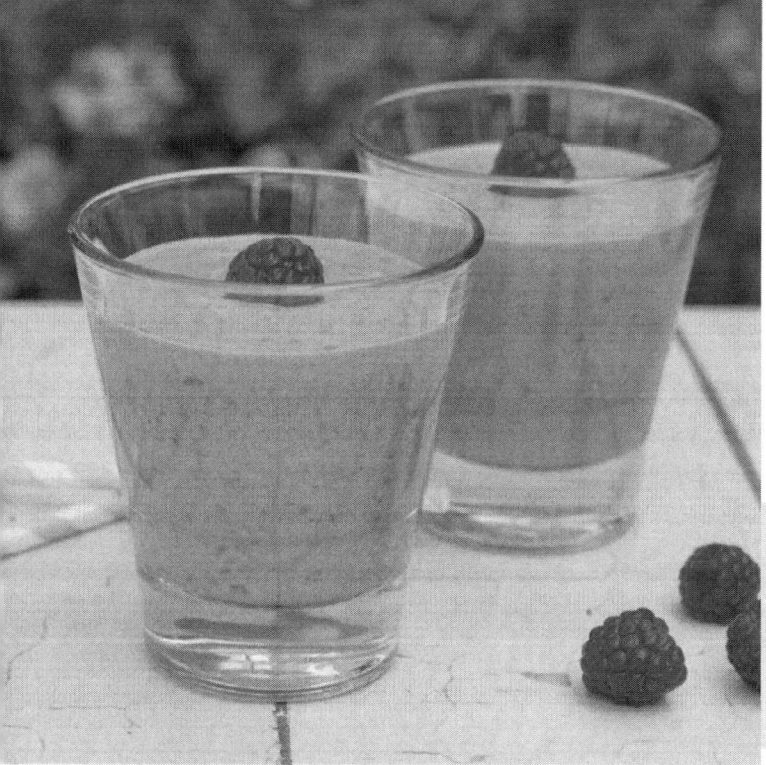

SMOOTHIES

RASPBERRY AND COCOA SMOOTHIE

Anti-Inflammatory Benefits:
Raspberries are rich in antioxidants and fiber, while unsweetened cocoa powder contains flavonoids that help reduce inflammation and support heart health.

PREP TIME: 5 MINS **COOK TIME:** 00 MINS **SERVING: 1** Portion Size: : 1 glass

INGREDIENTS

- 1/2 cup (75 g) fresh raspberries
- 1 cup (240 ml) almond milk
- 1 tbsp (7 g) unsweetened cocoa powder
- 1 tsp (5 ml) honey or maple syrup (optional for sweetness)

INSTRUCTIONS

1. Combine all ingredients in a blender.
2. Blend on full power until the ingredient's texture looks smooth and creamy. Adjust with almond milk for the desired consistency.
3. Pour into a glass and serve immediately.

 EQUIPMENT NEEDED:
Blender, measuring cups

 **NUTRITIONAL INFORMATION** (PER SERVING):

Calories: 100 kcal, Carbohydrates: 20 g, Protein: 2 g, Fat: 3 g, Fiber: 4 g

HEALTH BENEFITS:
Seasonal Produce Swap: Substitute raspberries with strawberries or blackberries when in season.
Dietary Substitutions: Skip the honey for a lower-sugar option.

LUNCHES/LIGHT BITES

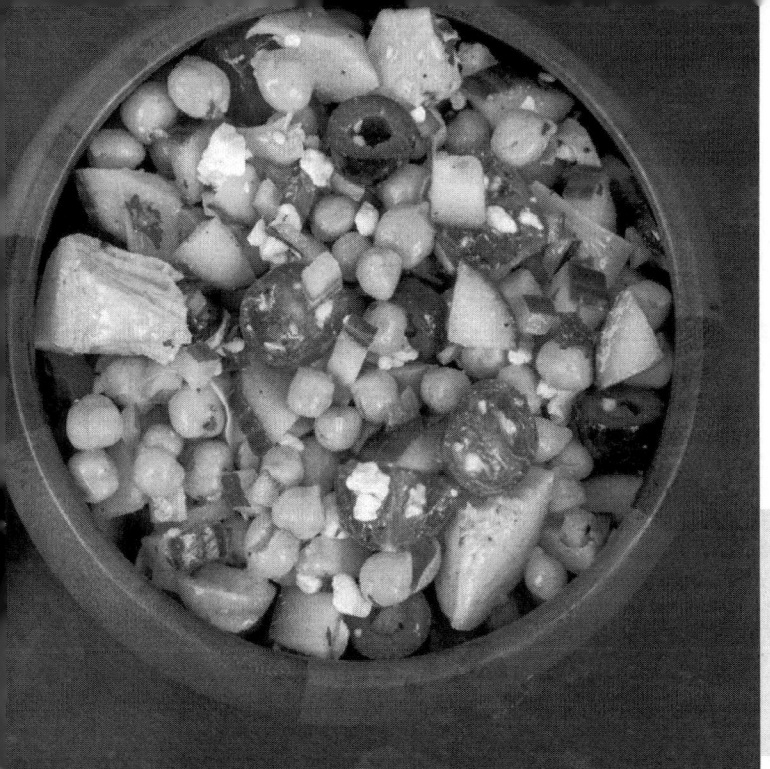

LUNCHES/LIGHT BITES

MEDITERRANEAN CHICKPEA SALAD WITH OLIVES

Anti-Inflammatory Benefits:
Chickpeas are high in fiber and protein, supporting gut health and reducing inflammation, while olives provide healthy fats that promote heart health.

PREP TIME: 10 MINS   **COOK TIME:** 00 MINS   **SERVING: 2** Portion Size: 1 bowl per serving

INGREDIENTS

- 1 cup (150 g) cooked chickpeas (canned or freshly cooked)
- 1/4 cup (40 g) Kalamata olives, sliced
- 1/2 cup (75 g) cherry tomatoes, halved
- 1/4 cucumber (50 g), diced
- 2 tbsp (30 ml) olive oil
- 1 tbsp (15 ml) lemon juice
- 1 tsp dried oregano
- Salt and pepper to taste

 EQUIPMENT NEEDED:

Mixing bowl, spoon

INSTRUCTIONS

1. Take a large, deep-bottom bowl and combine the chickpeas, olives, cherry tomatoes, and cucumber.
2. Drizzle two tbsp oil and lemon juice, then sprinkle with oregano, salt, and pepper.
3. Toss well to combine and serve immediately or refrigerate for up to 1 day.

 NUTRITIONAL INFORMATION (PER SERVING):

Calories: 220 kcal, Carbohydrates: 20 g, Protein: 6 g, Fat: 12 g, Fiber: 5 g

HEALTH BENEFITS:
Seasonal Produce Swap: Add fresh herbs like parsley or cilantro for additional flavor.
Dietary Substitutions: For a tangy twist, add crumbled feta cheese.

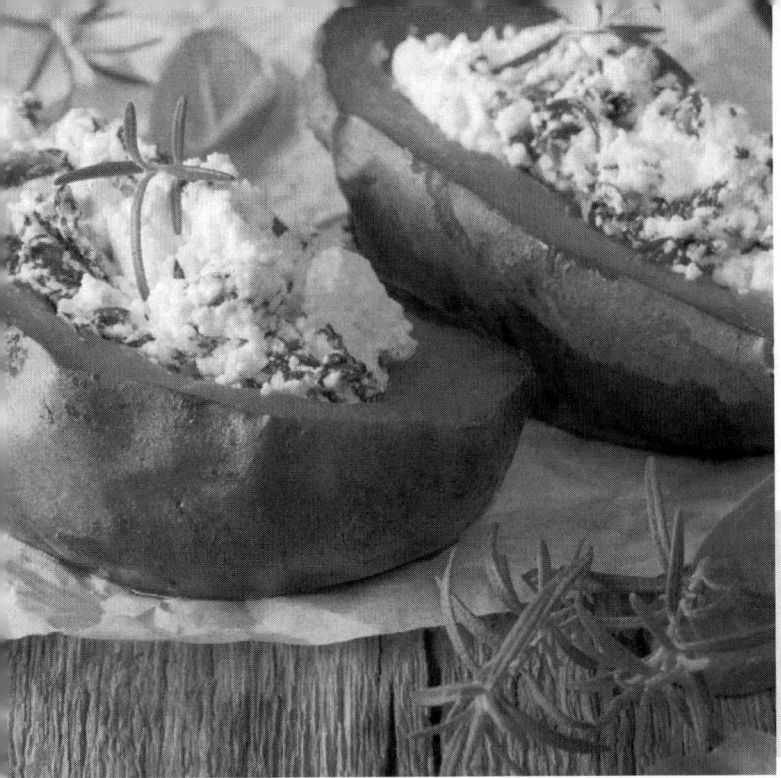

LUNCHES/LIGHT BITES

SPINACH AND FETA STUFFED SWEET POTATOES

Anti-Inflammatory Benefits:
Sweet potatoes are high in beta-carotene and fiber, which support immune health. Spinach provides anti-inflammatory vitamins, and feta adds a tangy flavor and protein boost.

PREP TIME: 10 MINS **COOK TIME:** 30 MINS **SERVING: 2** Portion Size: 1 stuffed sweet potato per serving

INGREDIENTS

- 2 medium sweet potatoes (300 g total)
- 1 cup (30 g) fresh spinach, chopped
- 1/4 cup (40 g) feta cheese, crumbled
- 1 tbsp (15 ml) olive oil
- 1/4 tsp (1 g) crushed black pepper

 EQUIPMENT NEEDED:
Baking sheet, knife, skillet

INSTRUCTIONS

1. Preheat oven to 400°F (200°C). Pierce the sweet potatoes, then spread them on the paper-arranged baking sheet and bake for 30 minutes or until tender.
2. While the sweet potatoes bake, heat one tbsp oil in a skillet over moderate stove flame and sauté the spinach until wilted.
3. Once done, cut them in half lengthwise and scoop out a small segment of the flesh to create a cavity.
4. Fill each sweet potato with the sautéed spinach and sprinkle with feta cheese.
5. Return to the oven for 5 minutes to warm the filling, then serve immediately.

 NUTRITIONAL INFORMATION (PER SERVING):

Calories: 200 kcal, Carbohydrates: 30 g, Protein: 5 g, Fat: 7 g, Fiber: 6 g

HEALTH BENEFITS:
Seasonal Produce Swap: Substitute spinach with kale or arugula.
Dietary Substitutions: Use dairy-free cheese for a vegan option.

32

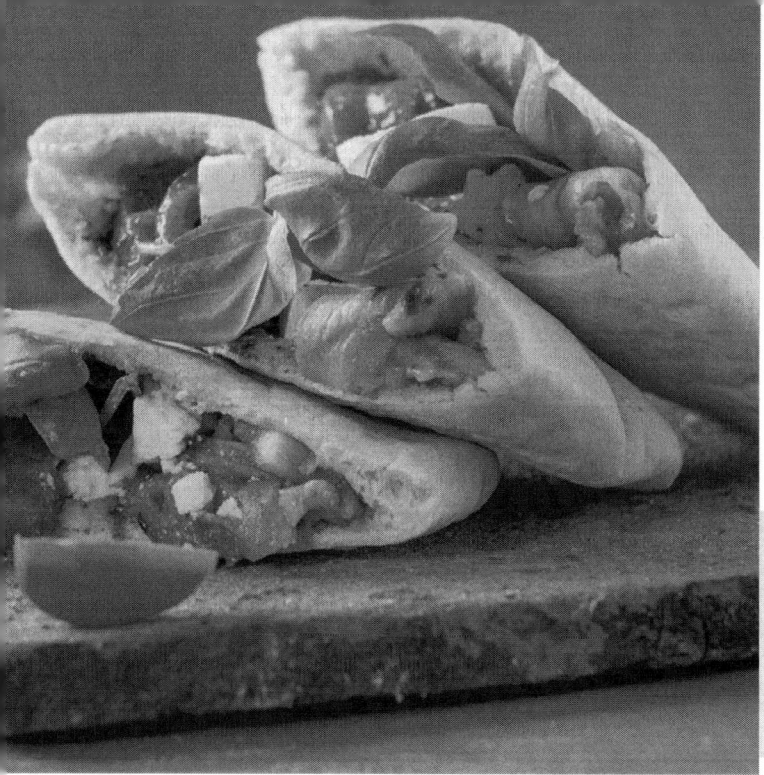

LUNCHES/LIGHT BITES

GRILLED VEGGIE PITA POCKET

Anti-Inflammatory Benefits:
Grilled vegetables like zucchini and bell peppers are rich in antioxidants that help reduce inflammation, while whole-grain pita adds fiber.

PREP TIME: 10 MINS   **COOK TIME:** 10 MINS   **SERVING: 2** Portion Size: 1 stuffed pita per serving

INGREDIENTS

- 1 medium zucchini (150 g), sliced
- 1/2 red bell pepper (50 g), sliced
- 1/4 cup (40 g) cherry tomatoes, halved
- 1/4 cup (60 g) hummus
- 2 whole-grain pita pockets

 EQUIPMENT NEEDED:
Grill pan or skillet, knife, spoon

INSTRUCTIONS

1. Heat a grill pan over moderate stove flame and grill the zucchini and bell pepper slices until tender, about 5 minutes.
2. Cut the pita pockets in half and spread 2 tbsp of hummus inside each half.
3. Stuff each pita half with grilled vegetables and cherry tomatoes.
4. Serve immediately.

 NUTRITIONAL INFORMATION (PER SERVING):

Calories: 220 kcal, Carbohydrates: 35 g, Protein: 6 g, Fat: 6 g, Fiber: 5 g

HEALTH BENEFITS:
Seasonal Produce Swap: Add grilled eggplant or mushrooms for variety.
Dietary Substitutions: Use gluten-free pita bread if needed.

33

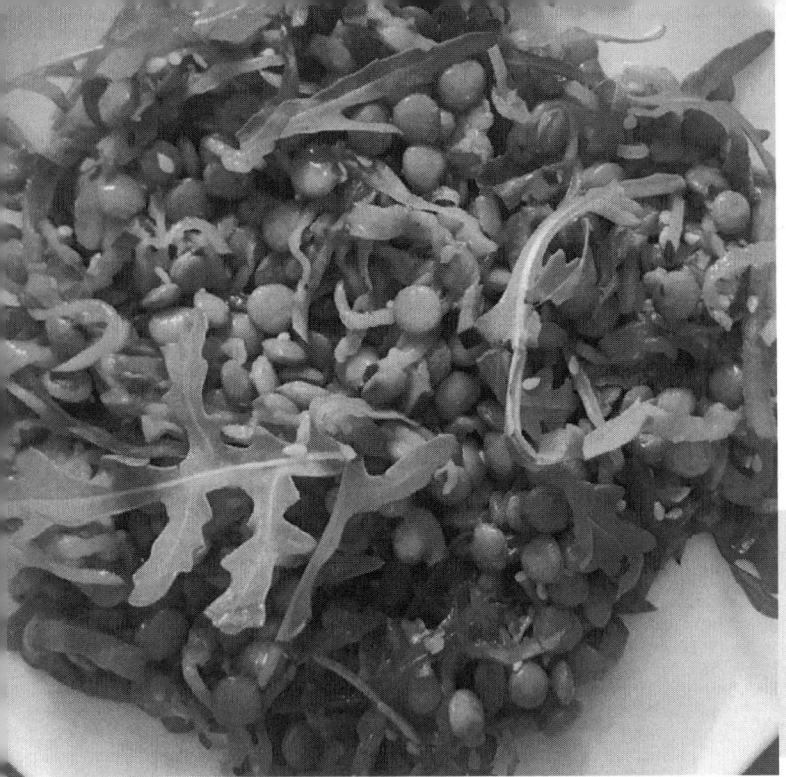

LUNCHES/LIGHT BITES

WARM LENTIL AND ARUGULA SALAD

Anti-Inflammatory Benefits:
Lentils are high in protein and fiber, promoting gut health and reducing inflammation. Arugula adds a peppery flavor and antioxidants.

PREP TIME: 10 MINS   **COOK TIME:** 15 MINS   **SERVING: 2** Portion Size: 1 bowl per serving

INGREDIENTS

- 1/2 cup (90 g) dry lentils
- 1 1/2 cups (360 ml) water
- 1 cup (30 g) fresh arugula
- 2 tbsp (30 ml) olive oil
- 1 tbsp (15 ml) balsamic vinegar
- Salt and pepper to taste

INSTRUCTIONS

1. Rinse the lentils and place them in a saucepan with water. Get it to a boil, then decrease the stove heat and simmer for 15 minutes or until tender. Drain and cool slightly.
2. Take a large deep-bottom bowl and combine the lentils, arugula, olive oil, and balsamic vinegar.
3. Powder it with salt and crushed pepper, toss well, and serve warm.

 EQUIPMENT NEEDED:
Saucepan, mixing bowl, spoon

 **NUTRITIONAL INFORMATION** (PER SERVING):

Calories: 180 kcal, Carbohydrates: 20 g, Protein: 8 g, Fat: 8 g, Fiber: 7 g

HEALTH BENEFITS:
Seasonal Produce Swap: Use baby spinach or mixed greens in place of arugula.
Dietary Substitutions: Add goat cheese for extra flavor.

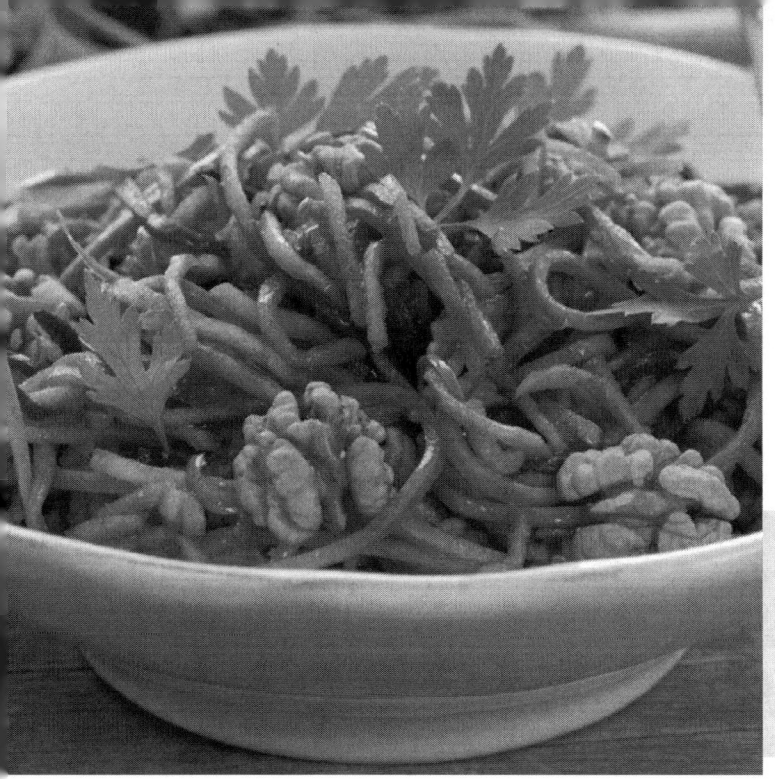

LUNCHES/LIGHT BITES

BEET AND CARROT SALAD WITH WALNUTS

Anti-Inflammatory Benefits:
Beets are high in antioxidants and nitrates that reduce inflammation, while carrots provide beta-carotene, and walnuts add omega-3 fatty acids.

PREP TIME: 10 MINS **COOK TIME:** 00 MINS **SERVING: 2** Portion Size: 1 bowl per serving

INGREDIENTS

- 1 medium beet (100 g), grated
- 1 medium carrot (50 g), grated
- 1/4 cup (30 g) walnuts, chopped
- 2 tbsp (30 ml) olive oil
- 1 tbsp (15 ml) lemon juice

INSTRUCTIONS

1. Take a large, deep-bottom bowl and combine the grated beet, grated carrot, and walnuts.
2. Drizzle two tbsp oil and lemon juice, then toss well.
3. Serve immediately.

 NUTRITIONAL INFORMATION (PER SERVING):

Calories: 170 kcal, Carbohydrates: 12 g, Protein: 3 g, Fat: 12 g, Fiber: 4 g

HEALTH BENEFITS:
Seasonal Produce Swap: Substitute walnuts with pecans or sunflower seeds.
Dietary Substitutions: Add crumbled goat cheese for a richer flavor.

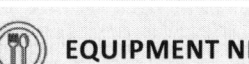 **EQUIPMENT NEEDED:**

Grater, mixing bowl

35

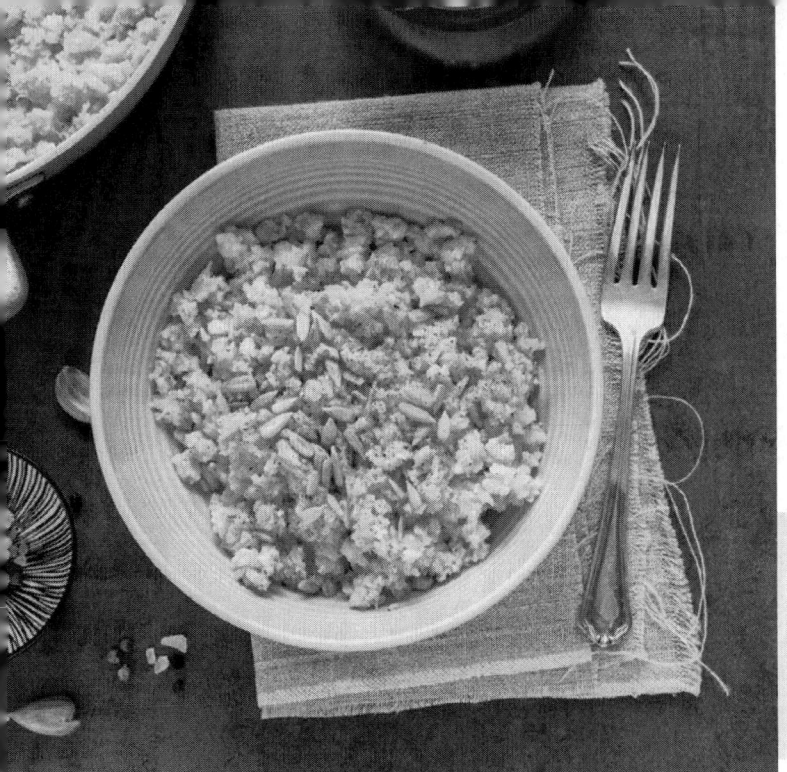

LUNCHES/LIGHT BITES

TURMERIC-SPICED CAULIFLOWER RICE BOWL

Anti-Inflammatory Benefits:
Cauliflower is a cruciferous vegetable rich in antioxidants and anti-inflammatory compounds, while turmeric contains curcumin, a powerful anti-inflammatory spice.

PREP TIME:
10 MINS

COOK TIME:
10 MINS

SERVING: 2
Portion Size: 1 bowl per serving

INGREDIENTS

- 2 cups (200 g) cauliflower rice (store-bought or freshly grated)
- 1/2 tsp (1 g) ground turmeric
- 1/2 cup (50 g) cooked chickpeas
- 1/4 cup (40 g) cherry tomatoes, halved
- 1/4 avocado (30 g), diced
- 1 tbsp (15 ml) olive oil
- Salt and pepper to taste

 EQUIPMENT NEEDED:

Skillet, knife, spatula

INSTRUCTIONS

1. Heat one tbsp oil in a skillet over moderate stove flame. Add cauliflower rice and turmeric, stirring to coat evenly.
2. Cook for 5–7 minutes until the veggies rice gets tender.
3. Divide the cauliflower rice into two bowls and top with chickpeas, cherry tomatoes, and diced avocado.
4. Powder it with salt and crushed pepper and serve warm.

 NUTRITIONAL INFORMATION (PER SERVING):

Calories: 180 kcal, Carbohydrates: 15 g, Protein: 6 g, Fat: 10 g, Fiber: 5 g

HEALTH BENEFITS:
Seasonal Produce Swap: Add fresh herbs like parsley or cilantro for extra flavor.
Dietary Substitutions: Substitute chickpeas with black beans for variety.

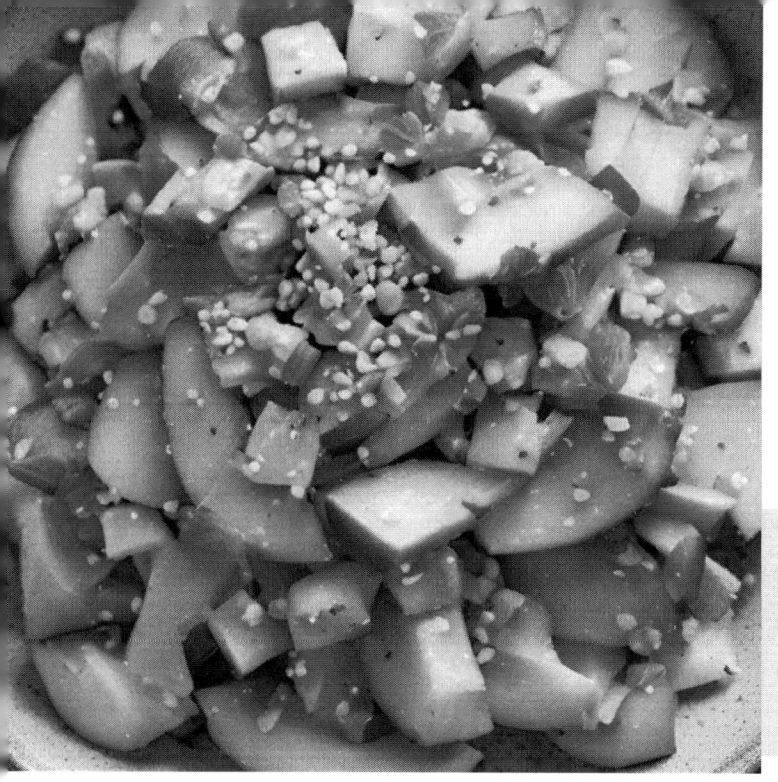

LUNCHES/LIGHT BITES

CUCUMBER AND AVOCADO SALAD WITH SESAME

Anti-Inflammatory Benefits:
Cucumbers are hydrating and contain anti-inflammatory compounds, while avocados provide healthy monounsaturated fats to reduce inflammation.

PREP TIME: 10 MINS

COOK TIME: 00 MINS

SERVING: 2
Portion Size: 1 bowl per serving

INGREDIENTS

- 1 medium cucumber (150 g), sliced
- 1/2 avocado (60 g), diced
- 1 tbsp (15 g) sesame seeds
- 1 tbsp (15 ml) lemon juice
- 1 tbsp (15 ml) olive oil
- Salt and pepper to taste

EQUIPMENT NEEDED:
Knife, mixing bowl

INSTRUCTIONS

1. Take a large, deep-bottom bowl and combine the cucumber slices and diced avocado.
2. Drizzle lemon juice and one tbsp oil, then sprinkle with sesame seeds, salt, and pepper.
3. Toss gently and serve immediately.

NUTRITIONAL INFORMATION (PER SERVING):

Calories: 140 kcal, Carbohydrates: 6 g, Protein: 2 g, Fat: 12 g, Fiber: 4 g

HEALTH BENEFITS:
Seasonal Produce Swap: Use zucchini slices instead of cucumber during summer.
Dietary Substitutions: Add sunflower seeds instead of sesame for a nut-free option.

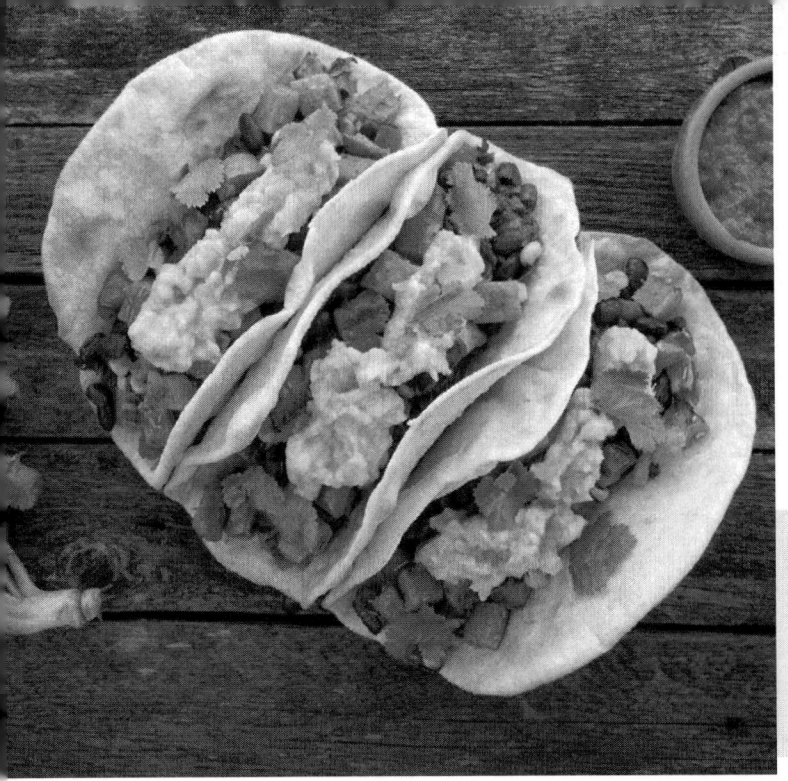

LUNCHES/LIGHT BITES

SWEET POTATO AND BLACK BEAN TACOS

Anti-Inflammatory Benefits:
Sweet potatoes provide beta-carotene and fiber, while black beans are a great source of plant-based protein and antioxidants.

PREP TIME: 10 MINS

COOK TIME: 20 MINS

SERVING: 4
Portion Size: 2 tacos per serving

INGREDIENTS

- 1 medium sweet potato (150 g), diced
- 1 cup (150 g) black beans (canned or cooked)
- 4 small corn tortillas
- 1/4 cup (40 g) cherry tomatoes, diced
- 1/4 avocado (30 g), sliced
- 1 tbsp (15 ml) olive oil
- 1/2 tsp (1 g) ground cumin
- Salt and pepper to taste

EQUIPMENT NEEDED:
Baking sheet, skillet, spatula

INSTRUCTIONS

1. Preheat oven to 400°F (200°C). Toss the sweet potato wedges with olive oil, cumin, salt, and pepper, then spread on a baking sheet. Roast for 20 minutes until tender.
2. Warm the tortillas over low heat.
3. Fill each tortilla with roasted sweet potatoes, black beans, cherry tomatoes, and avocado slices.
4. Serve immediately.

NUTRITIONAL INFORMATION (PER SERVING):

Calories: 250 kcal, Carbohydrates: 38 g, Protein: 6 g, Fat: 8 g, Fiber: 8 g

HEALTH BENEFITS:
Seasonal Produce Swap: Add fresh corn or diced zucchini in summer. Add fresh corn or diced zucchini in summer.
Dietary Substitutions: Use whole-grain tortillas for added fiber.

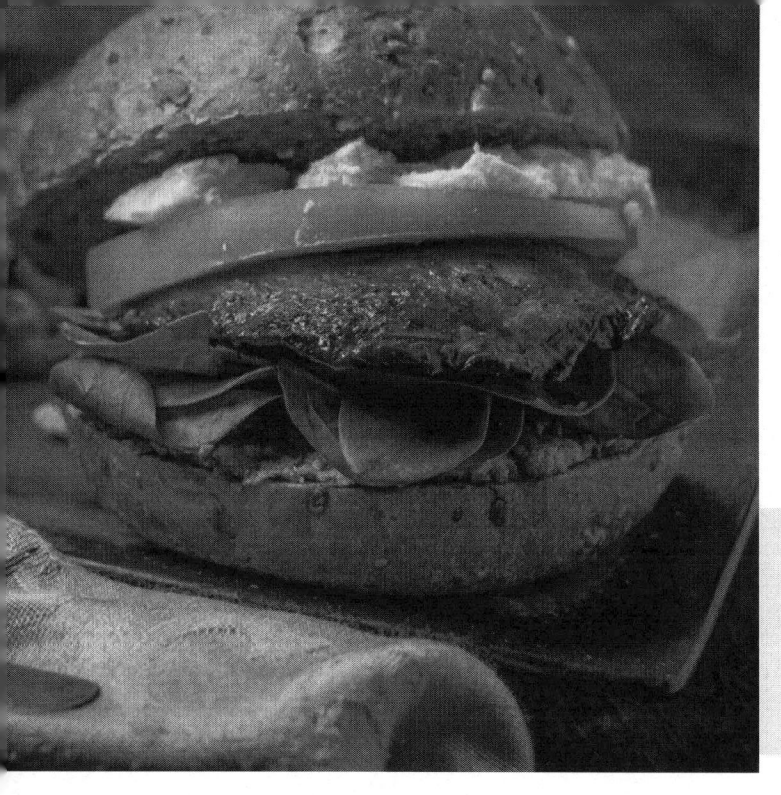

LUNCHES/LIGHT BITES

GRILLED PORTOBELLO MUSHROOM SANDWICH

Anti-Inflammatory Benefits:
Portobello mushrooms are rich in antioxidants and anti-inflammatory compounds, while whole-grain bread adds fiber for gut health.

PREP TIME: 10 MINS

COOK TIME: 10 MINS

SERVING: 2
Portion Size: 1 sandwich per serving

INGREDIENTS

- 2 large Portobello mushrooms (150 g total), stems removed
- 1 tbsp (15 ml) balsamic vinegar
- 1 tbsp (15 ml) olive oil
- 2 slices whole-grain bread
- 1/4 cup (40 g) hummus
- 1/4 cup (30 g) fresh spinach leaves

EQUIPMENT NEEDED:
Grill pan, spatula, knife

INSTRUCTIONS

1. Preheat grill pan over moderate stove flame. Drizzle the mushrooms with balsamic vinegar and olive oil.
2. Grill the mushrooms for 5 minutes on one side or until tender and slightly charred.
3. Toast the whole-grain bread slices. Spread hummus on each slice, then layer with grilled mushrooms and fresh spinach.
4. Assemble the sandwich and serve warm.

NUTRITIONAL INFORMATION (PER SERVING):

Calories: 220 kcal, Carbohydrates: 26 g, Protein: 6 g, Fat: 10 g, Fiber: 5 g

HEALTH BENEFITS:
Seasonal Produce Swap: Add grilled zucchini or bell peppers for extra flavor.
Dietary Substitutions: Use gluten-free bread if needed.

DINNERS

DINNERS

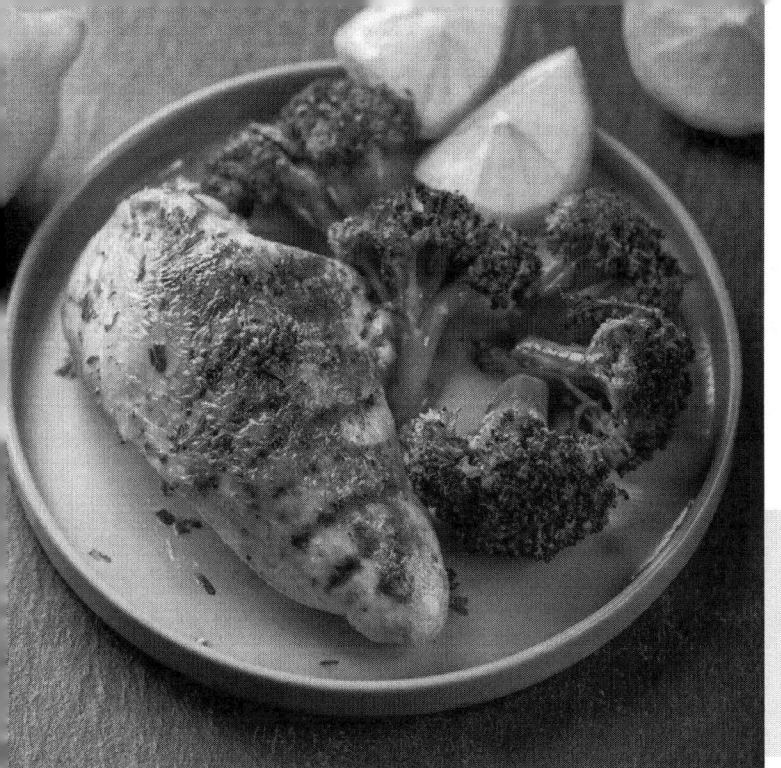

GRILLED LEMON HERB CHICKEN WITH BROCCOLI

Anti-Inflammatory Benefits:
Chicken provides lean protein to support muscle repair, while broccoli is high in antioxidants and anti-inflammatory nutrients like sulforaphane.

PREP TIME: 10 MINS

COOK TIME: 20 MINS

SERVING: 3
Portion Size: 1 chicken breast and 1 cup of broccoli per serving

INGREDIENTS

- 3 boneless, skinless chicken breasts (500 g total)
- 1 medium lemon (50 ml juice), juiced
- 2 tsp (5 g) dried Italian herbs
- 1 tbsp (15 ml) olive oil
- 3 cups (300 g) broccoli florets
- Salt and pepper to taste

EQUIPMENT NEEDED:
Grill pan, skillet, knife, mixing bowl

INSTRUCTIONS

1. Take a large deep-bottom bowl and combine the lemon juice, Italian herbs, olive oil, salt, and pepper. Add breast meat and marinate for at least 10 minutes.
2. Heat a grill pan over moderate stove flame. Cook the breast meat for 6–8 minutes on one side until fully cooked.
3. In a skillet, steam or sauté the broccoli with a small amount of water until tender, about 5 minutes.
4. Serve each chicken breast with a side of broccoli.

NUTRITIONAL INFORMATION (PER SERVING):

Calories: 240 kcal, Carbohydrates: 8 g, Protein: 30 g, Fat: 8 g, Fiber: 3 g

HEALTH BENEFITS:
Seasonal Produce Swap: Substitute broccoli with green beans or asparagus.
Dietary Substitutions: Use tofu as a plant-based alternative.

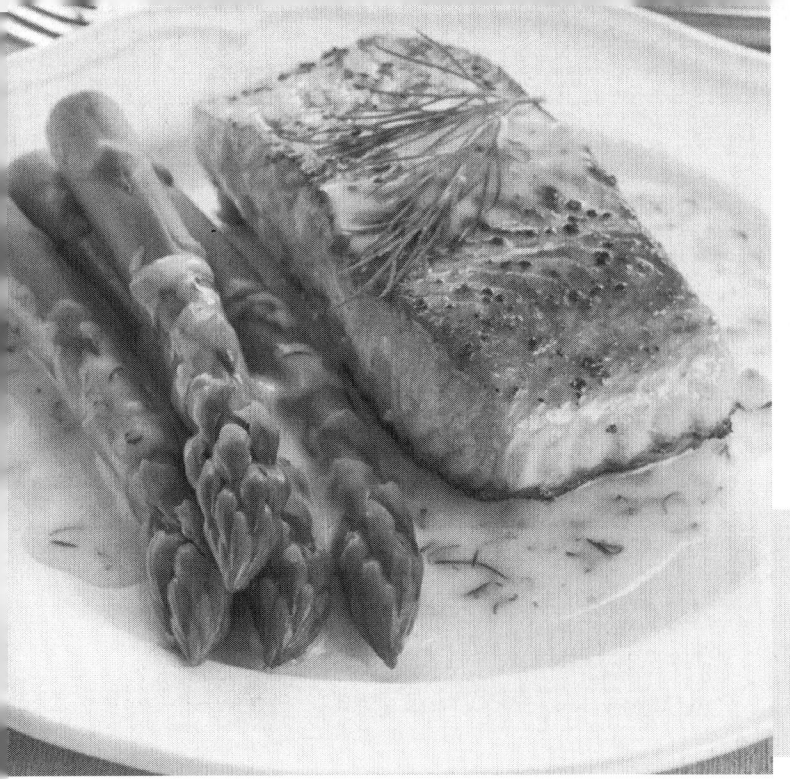

BAKED SALMON WITH ASPARAGUS AND LEMON

DINNERS

Anti-Inflammatory Benefits:
Salmon is rich in omega-3 fatty acids, which reduce inflammation, while asparagus contains anti-inflammatory compounds and antioxidants.

PREP TIME: 10 MINS

COOK TIME: 15 MINS

SERVING: 2
Portion Size: 1 salmon fillet and 1 cup of asparagus per serving

INGREDIENTS

- 2 salmon fillets (300 g total)
- 1 cup (150 g) asparagus spears, trimmed
- 1 tbsp (15 ml) olive oil
- 1/2 lemon (25 ml juice), juiced
- Salt and pepper to taste

EQUIPMENT NEEDED:
Baking sheet, aluminum foil, knife

INSTRUCTIONS

1. Preheat oven to 375°F (190°C). Arrange the baking sheet with aluminum foil.
2. Place the salmon fillets and asparagus on the paper-arranged baking sheet. Drizzle one tbsp oil and lemon juice, then powder it with salt and crushed pepper.
3. Fold the foil around the salmon and asparagus to create a sealed packet.
4. Bake for 12–15 minutes, or until the salmon is done throughly and flakes easily with a fork.
5. Serve immediately.

NUTRITIONAL INFORMATION (PER SERVING):

Calories: 280 kcal, Carbohydrates: 4 g, Protein: 30 g, Fat: 15 g, Fiber: 2 g

HEALTH BENEFITS:
Seasonal Produce Swap: Use green beans or zucchini instead of asparagus.
Dietary Substitutions: For a vegetarian option, replace salmon with tofu or tempeh.

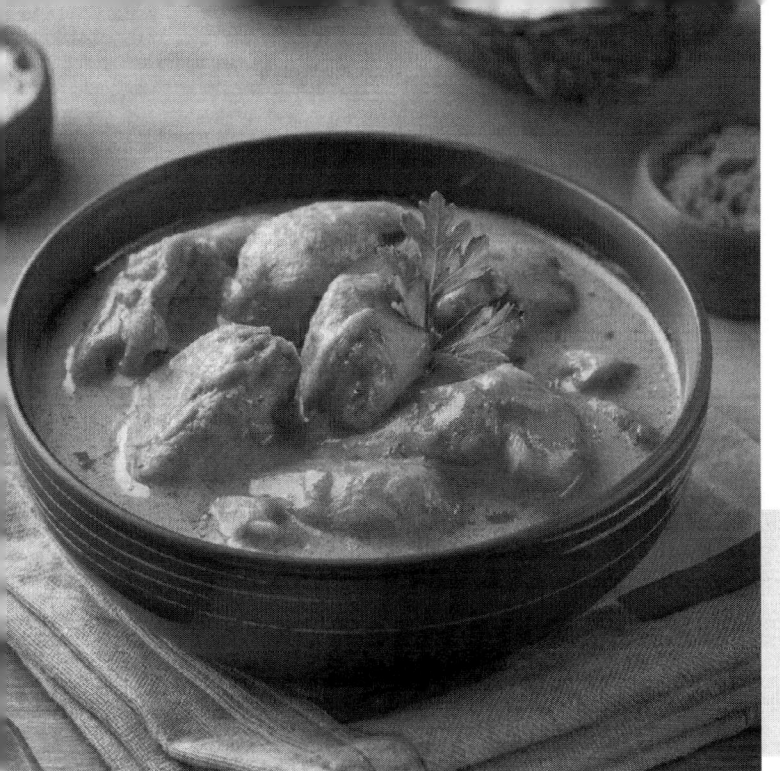

TURMERIC-COCONUT CHICKEN CURRY

DINNERS

Anti-Inflammatory Benefits:
Turmeric contains curcumin, a powerful anti-inflammatory compound, while coconut milk adds healthy fats to support gut and brain health.

PREP TIME: 15 MINS

COOK TIME: 25 MINS

SERVING: 3
Portion Size: 1 bowl per serving broccoli per serving

INGREDIENTS

- 2 boneless, skinless chicken thighs (300 g), diced
- 1 cup (240 ml) coconut milk
- 1 cup (100 g) diced sweet potato
- 1/2 cup (75 g) diced onion
- 1/2 tsp (1 g) ground turmeric
- 1 tbsp (15 ml) olive oil
- 1/2 tsp (1 g) ground ginger
- Salt to taste

EQUIPMENT NEEDED:
Large pot or skillet, knife

INSTRUCTIONS

1. Heat one tbsp oil in a pot or skillet over moderate stove flame. Add meat pieces and cook until browned about 5 minutes.
2. Add chopped onion, turmeric, and ginger. Cook for another 2 minutes until fragrant.
3. Toss in the sweet potato and coconut milk. Bring to a simmer and cover.
4. Cook for 15–20 minutes, keep stirring occasionally, until the chicken is done properly and the sweet potato is tender.
5. Serve warm.

NUTRITIONAL INFORMATION (PER SERVING):

Calories: 290 kcal, Carbohydrates: 10 g, Protein: 22 g, Fat: 18 g, Fiber: 2 g

HEALTH BENEFITS:
Seasonal Produce Swap: Replace sweet potato with butternut squash or carrots.
Dietary Substitutions: Use chickpeas instead of chicken for a vegan option.

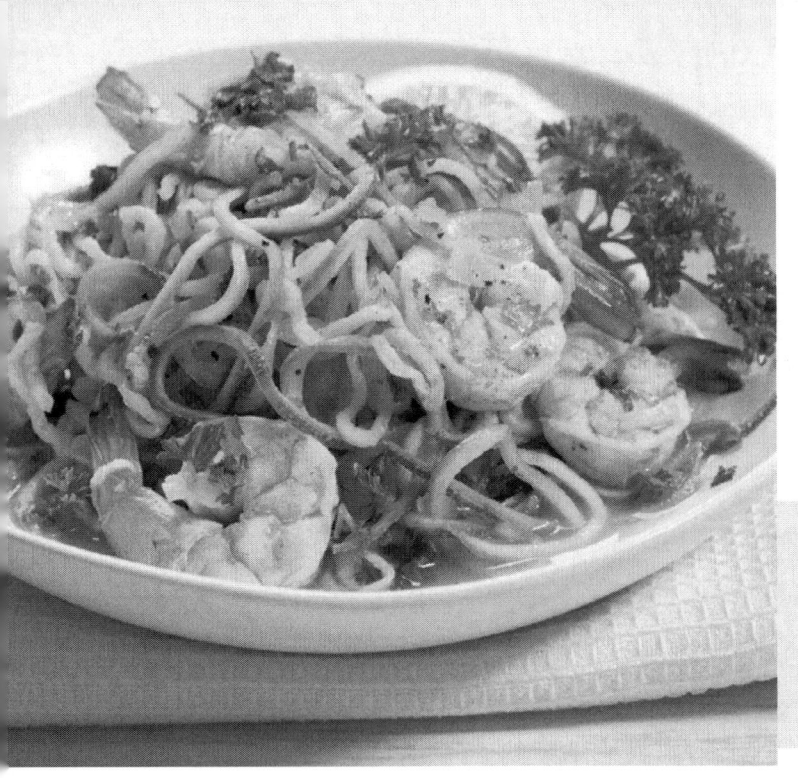

SHRIMP AND ZUCCHINI NOODLES WITH GARLIC

DINNERS

Anti-Inflammatory Benefits:
Shrimp provides lean protein, while zucchini noodles are low in calories and packed with antioxidants.

PREP TIME: 10 MINS

COOK TIME: 10 MINS

SERVING: 2
Portion Size: 1 bowl per serving

INGREDIENTS

- 2 medium zucchinis (300 g), spiralized
- 200 g raw shrimp, peeled and deveined
- 2 cloves garlic, minced
- 1 tbsp (15 ml) olive oil
- Salt and pepper to taste

EQUIPMENT NEEDED:
Spiralizer or julienne peeler, skillet, spatula

INSTRUCTIONS

1. Heat one tbsp oil in a skillet over moderate stove flame. Add garlic and sauté for 1 minute.
2. Add shrimp and sear for 3 minutes on one side until pink and fully cooked.
3. Toss in zucchini noodles and cook for 2 minutes, stirring occasionally.
4. Powder it with salt and crushed pepper and serve immediately.

NUTRITIONAL INFORMATION (PER SERVING):

Calories: 180 kcal, Carbohydrates: 6 g, Protein: 20 g, Fat: 8 g, Fiber: 2 g

HEALTH BENEFITS:
Seasonal Produce Swap: Use spaghetti squash in place of zucchini noodles.
Dietary Substitutions: Replace shrimp with tofu for a vegan option.

DINNERS

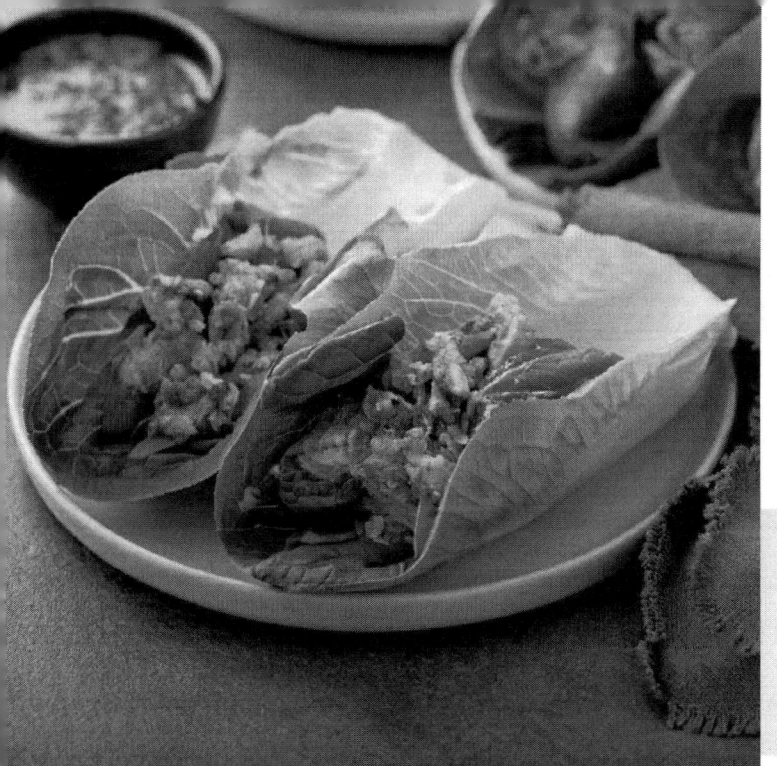

THAI BASIL TURKEY LETTUCE WRAPS

Anti-Inflammatory Benefits:
Ground turkey is a lean protein source, while fresh basil contains anti-inflammatory essential oils and antioxidants.

PREP TIME: 10 MINS
COOK TIME: 15 MINS
SERVING: 2 Portion 3 wraps per serving

INGREDIENTS

- 200 g ground turkey
- 6 large lettuce leaves
- 1/2 cup (75 g) diced bell peppers
- 2 tbsp (30 ml) soy sauce (low sodium)
- 1 tbsp (15 ml) olive oil
- 1/4 cup (10 g) basil leaves, chopped

EQUIPMENT NEEDED:
Skillet, spatula

INSTRUCTIONS

1. Heat one tbsp oil in a skillet over moderate stove flame. Add minced meat and cook until browned about 8–10 minutes.
2. Toss in the bell peppers, soy sauce, and basil, and cook for more 2–3 minutes.
3. Spoon the meat mixture over lettuce leaves in smooth way and serve immediately.

NUTRITIONAL INFORMATION (PER SERVING):

Calories: 200 kcal, Carbohydrates: 5 g, Protein: 25 g, Fat: 9 g, Fiber: 1 g

HEALTH BENEFITS:
Seasonal Produce Swap: Add diced zucchini or shredded carrots for extra vegetables.
Dietary Substitutions: Use tofu crumbles for a vegan version.

DINNERS

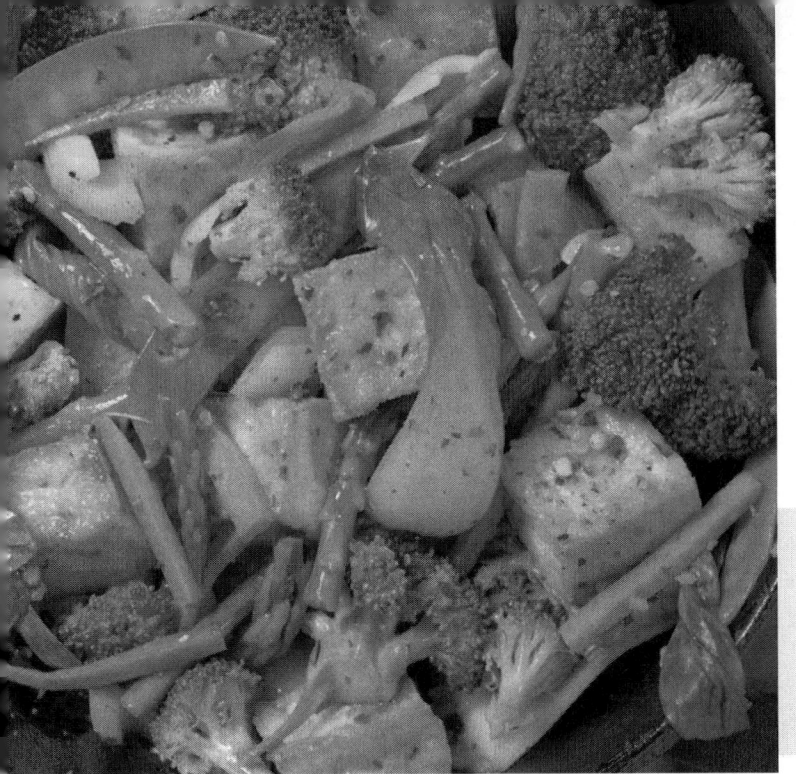

ROASTED VEGETABLE STIR-FRY WITH TOFU

Anti-Inflammatory Benefits:
Tofu is a great source of plant-based protein and anti-inflammatory isoflavones. Vegetables like bell peppers and broccoli are rich in antioxidants and vitamins.

PREP TIME: 10 MINS

COOK TIME: 20 MINS

SERVING: 3
Portion Size: 1 bowl per serving

INGREDIENTS

- 200 g firm tofu, cubed
- 1 cup (100 g) broccoli florets
- 1/2 red bell pepper (50 g), sliced
- 1/2 zucchini (50 g), sliced
- 1/2 cup (50 g) carrots, julienned
- 2 tbsp (30 ml) soy sauce (low-sodium)
- 1 tbsp (15 ml) olive oil
- 1 tsp grated ginger

EQUIPMENT NEEDED:
Skillet or wok, knife, spatula

INSTRUCTIONS

1. Heat one tbsp oil in a skillet or wok over moderate stove flame. Add tofu pieces and cook on all sides, about 5–7 minutes. Remove and set aside.
2. Add broccoli, bell pepper, zucchini, and carrots to the skillet. Stir-fry for 5–7 minutes until tender-crisp.
3. Toss in the soy sauce and ginger, then return the tofu to the skillet. Toss well to combine and cook for another 2 minutes.
4. Serve immediately.

NUTRITIONAL INFORMATION (PER SERVING):

Calories: 180 kcal, Carbohydrates: 12 g, Protein: 10 g, Fat: 10 g, Fiber: 4 g

HEALTH BENEFITS:
Seasonal Produce Swap: Use cauliflower or snap peas instead of broccoli.
Dietary Substitutions: Replace soy sauce with tamari for a gluten-free option.

DINNERS

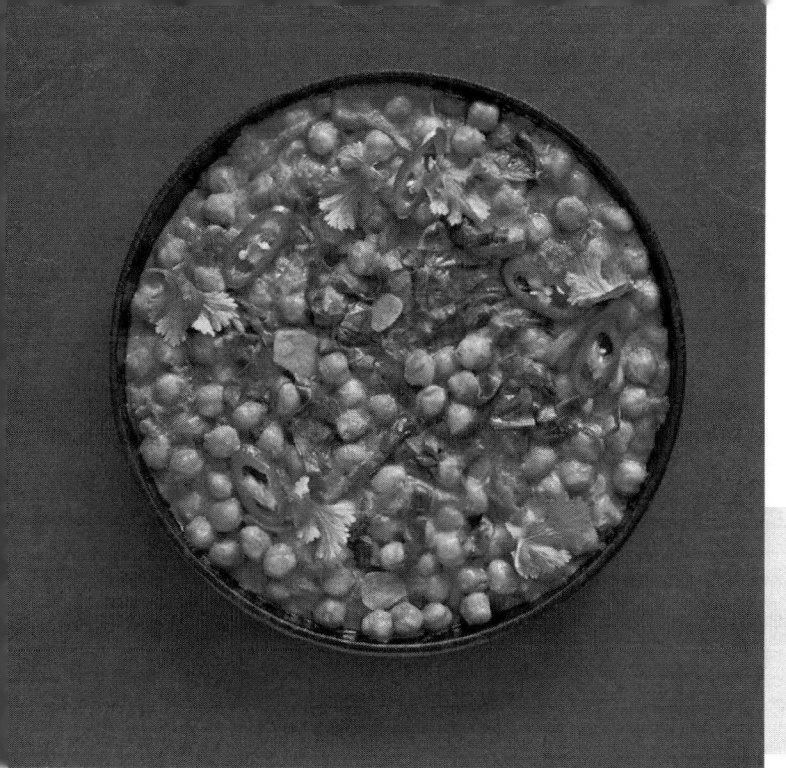

SPINACH AND CHICKPEA CURRY

Anti-Inflammatory Benefits:
Spinach is packed with anti-inflammatory nutrients like vitamin K, while chickpeas provide fiber and protein to support gut health.

PREP TIME: 10 MINS

COOK TIME: 20 MINS

SERVING: 3
Portion 1 bowl per serving

INGREDIENTS

- 1 cup (150 g) cooked chickpeas
- 2 cups (60 g) fresh spinach, chopped
- 1/2 cup (120 ml) coconut milk
- 1/2 cup (100 g) diced tomatoes
- 1/2 onion (50 g), diced
- 1 tsp (2 g) ground turmeric
- 1/2 tsp (1 g) ground cumin
- 1 tbsp (15 ml) olive oil

INSTRUCTIONS

1. Heat one tbsp oil in a pot or skillet over moderate stove flame. Add chopped onion and softened until soft, about 3 minutes.
2. Toss in the turmeric and cumin, and cook for 1 minute until fragrant.
3. Add diced tomatoes, chickpeas, and coconut milk. Simmer for 10 minutes.
4. Toss in spinach and cook for more 5 minutes, until wilted.
5. Serve warm.

EQUIPMENT NEEDED:
Pot or skillet, spoon

NUTRITIONAL INFORMATION (PER SERVING):

Calories: 220 kcal, Carbohydrates: 20 g, Protein: 7 g, Fat: 12 g, Fiber: 5 g

HEALTH BENEFITS:
Seasonal Produce Swap: Use kale or Swiss chard instead of spinach.
Dietary Substitutions: Replace chickpeas with lentils for variety.

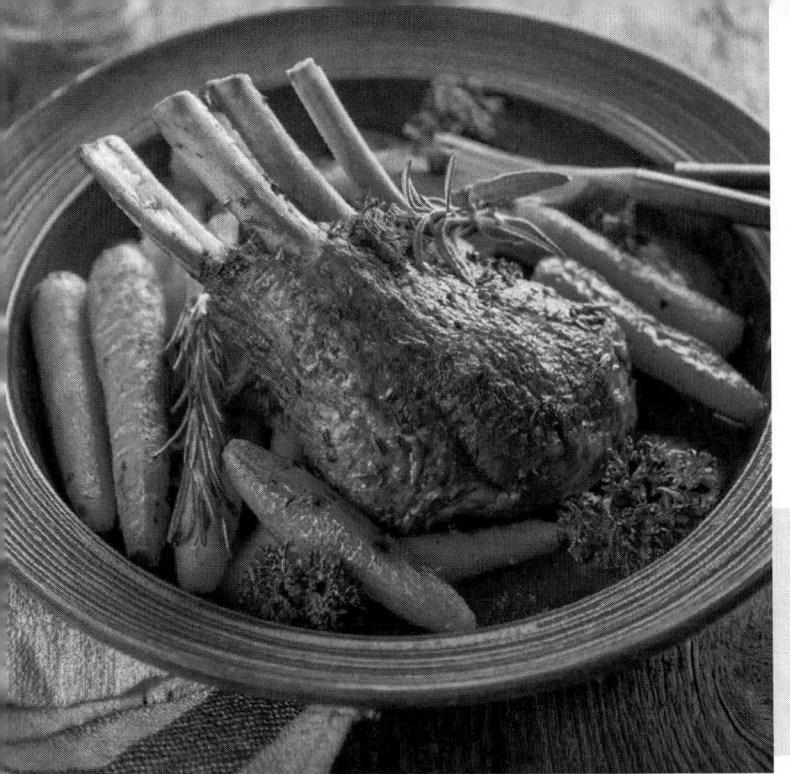

GARLIC AND HERB ROASTED LAMB WITH CARROTS

DINNERS

Anti-Inflammatory Benefits:
Lamb provides high-quality protein, while carrots are rich in beta-carotene and antioxidants, supporting immune and skin health.

PREP TIME: 15 MINS

COOK TIME: 35 MINS

SERVING: 3
Portion Size: 1 portion of lamb and 1 cup of carrots per serving

INGREDIENTS

- 400 g lamb loin chops
- 2 cups (200 g) carrots, peeled and sliced
- 1 tbsp (15 ml) olive oil
- 2 cloves garlic, minced
- 1 tsp (2 g) dried rosemary
- Salt and pepper to taste

EQUIPMENT NEEDED:
Skillet or wok, knife, spatula

INSTRUCTIONS

1. Preheat oven to 400°F (200°C). Arrange the baking sheet with parchment paper.
2. Take a large deep-bottom bowl and combine the olive oil, garlic, rosemary, salt, and pepper. Rub this mixture over the lamb chops.
3. Arrange the lamb chops and carrots on the paper-arranged baking sheet. Drizzle the carrots with some olive oil.
4. Roast for 30–35 minutes, flipping the lamb chops halfway through, until the lamb is cooked to your preferred doneness.
5. Serve warm.

NUTRITIONAL INFORMATION (PER SERVING):
Calories: 300 kcal, Carbohydrates: 10 g, Protein: 25 g, Fat: 15 g, Fiber: 3 g

HEALTH BENEFITS:
Seasonal Produce Swap: Use parsnips or turnips instead of carrots.
Dietary Substitutions: Replace lamb with chicken thighs for a lighter option.

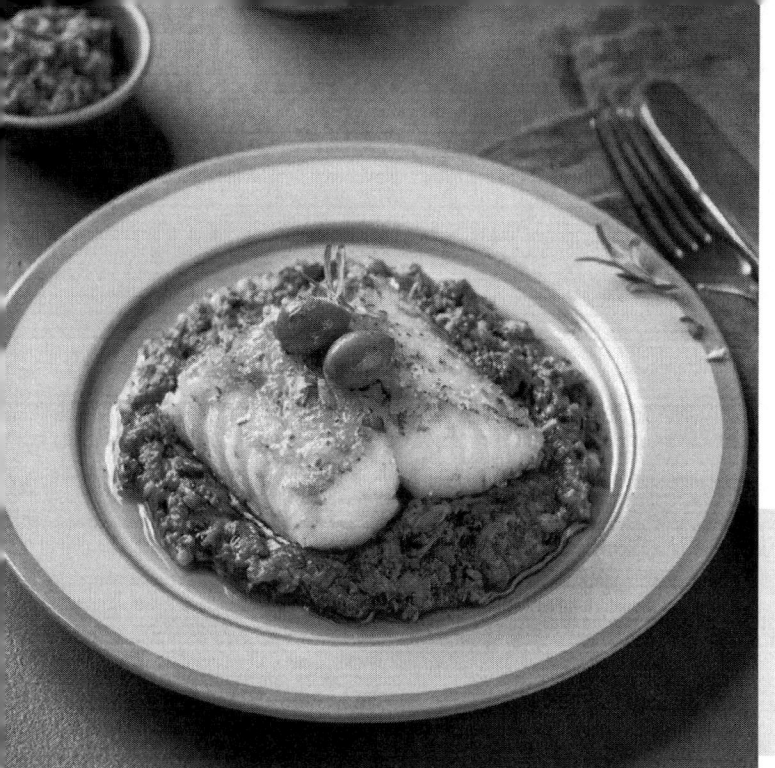

MEDITERRANEAN COD WITH OLIVE TAPENADE

DINNERS

Anti-Inflammatory Benefits:
Cod is a lean protein rich in anti-inflammatory omega-3 fatty acids, and olives provide heart-healthy monounsaturated fats.

PREP TIME: 10 MINS

COOK TIME: 15 MINS

SERVING: 2
Portion 1 cod fillet per serving

INGREDIENTS

- 2 cod fillets (300 g total)
- 1/4 cup (40 g) Kalamata olives, pitted
- 1 tbsp (15 ml) olive oil
- 1 tbsp (15 ml) lemon juice
- 1/2 tsp dried oregano

EQUIPMENT NEEDED:

Baking dish, food processor (optional)

INSTRUCTIONS

1. Preheat oven to 375°F (190°C).
2. Place the fish fillet fillets in a baking dish. Drizzle one tbsp oil and lemon juice, and sprinkle with oregano.
3. In a food processor or by hand, chop the Kalamata olives to create a coarse tapenade.
4. Spread the olive tapenade over the cod fillets.
5. Bake for 12–15 minutes until the cod flakes easily with a fork. Serve immediately.

NUTRITIONAL INFORMATION (PER SERVING):

Calories: 200 kcal, Carbohydrates: 2 g, Protein: 30 g, Fat: 8 g, Fiber: 1 g

HEALTH BENEFITS:

Seasonal Produce Swap: Serve with steamed asparagus or sautéed spinach as a side.
Dietary Substitutions: Use tofu or tempeh as a plant-based alternative.

BUDGET-FRIENDLY RECIPES

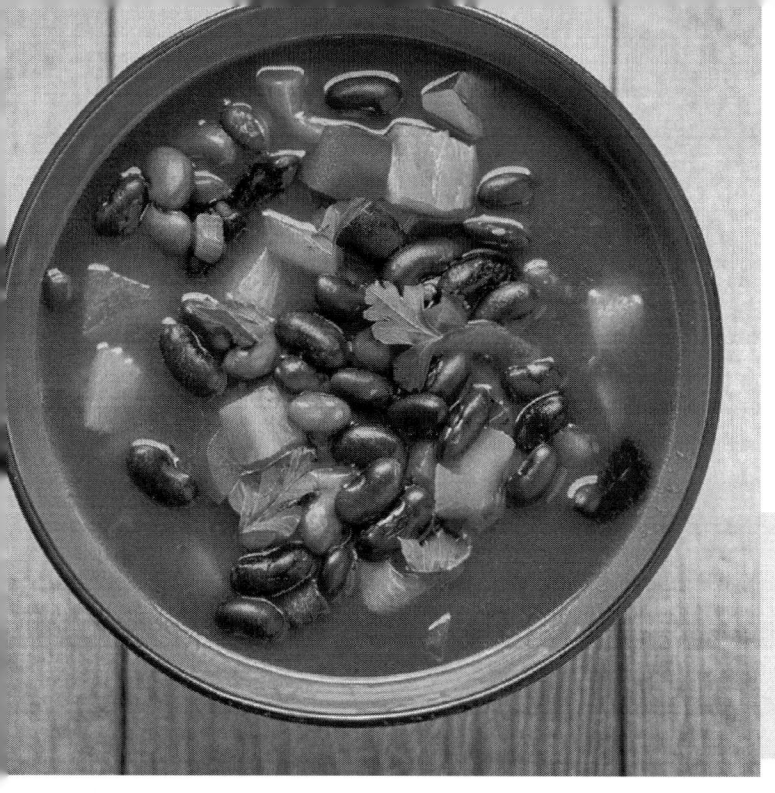

BUDGET-FRIENDLY RECIPES

BLACK BEAN AND VEGETABLE SOUP

Anti-Inflammatory Benefits:
Black beans are high in antioxidants and fiber, while vegetables like bell peppers and tomatoes provide vitamins and minerals that reduce inflammation.

PREP TIME: 10 MINS

COOK TIME: 20 MINS

SERVING: 4
Portion Size: 1 bowl per servings per serving

INGREDIENTS

- 1 cup (150 g) cooked black beans (or canned, drained and rinsed)
- 1/2 cup (75 g) diced tomatoes
- 1/2 cup (50 g) diced red bell pepper
- 1/2 cup (50 g) diced zucchini
- 1/4 cup (30 g) diced onion
- 2 cups (480 ml) vegetable broth
- 1 tsp (2 g) ground cumin
- Salt and pepper to taste

EQUIPMENT NEEDED:
Large pot, spoon

INSTRUCTIONS

1. Heat a small amount of oil in a pot over a moderate stove flame. Add chopped onion and bell pepper, and sauté for 3 minutes.
2. Add zucchini, tomatoes, black beans, and cumin. Stir well.
3. Pour in the vegetable broth and get it to a boil. Decrease the stove heat and simmer for 15 minutes.
4. Powder it with salt and crushed pepper, then serve warm.

NUTRITIONAL INFORMATION (PER SERVING):
Calories: 120 kcal, Carbohydrates: 18 g, Protein: 5 g, Fat: 2 g, Fiber: 6 g

HEALTH BENEFITS:
Seasonal Produce Swap: Use butternut squash or carrots instead of zucchini in the fall.
Dietary Substitutions: Add quinoa for extra protein and fiber.

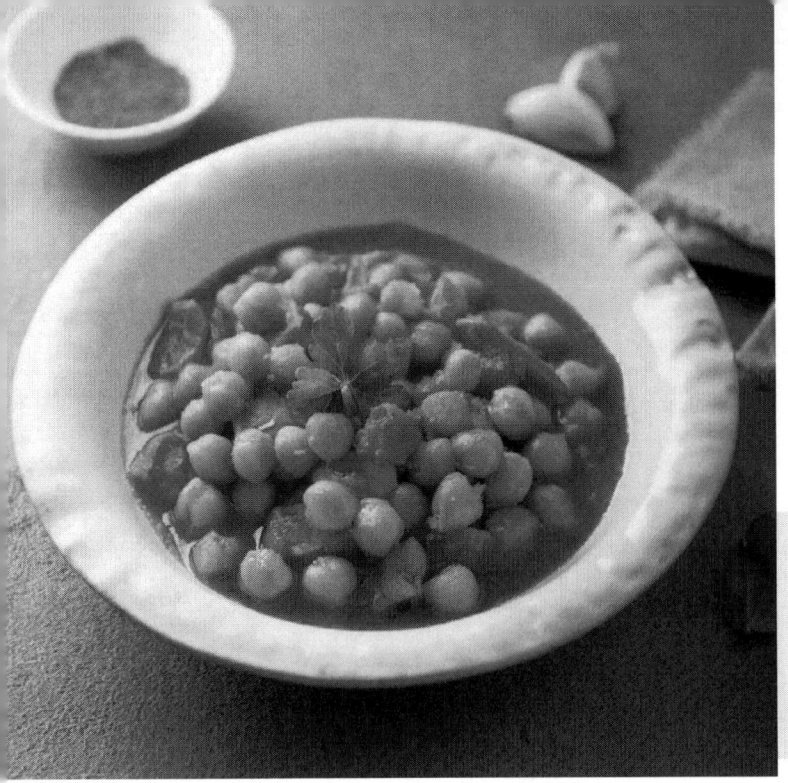

BUDGET-FRIENDLY RECIPES

CHICKPEA AND TOMATO STEW

Anti-Inflammatory Benefits:
Chickpeas are rich in plant-based protein and fiber, while tomatoes contain lycopene, a powerful antioxidant that reduces inflammation.

PREP TIME: 10 MINS

COOK TIME: 20 MINS

SERVING: 3
Portion Size: 1 bowl per serving per serving

INGREDIENTS

- 1 cup (150 g) cooked chickpeas (or canned, drained and rinsed)
- 1/2 cup (75 g) diced tomatoes
- 1/2 cup (50 g) diced carrots
- 1/2 cup (50 g) diced zucchini
- 1 cup (240 ml) vegetable broth
- 1/2 tsp (1 g) ground turmeric
- 1 tsp (2 g) ground cumin

EQUIPMENT NEEDED:
Pot, spoon

INSTRUCTIONS

1. Heat a small amount of oil in a pot over a moderate stove flame. Add carrots and cook for 3 minutes.
2. Add zucchini, chickpeas, tomatoes, turmeric, and cumin. Stir well.
3. Ladle in vegetable broth and simmer for 15 minutes.
4. Serve warm with fresh parsley on top if desired.

NUTRITIONAL INFORMATION (PER SERVING):

Calories: 150 kcal, Carbohydrates: 25 g, Protein: 6 g, Fat: 3 g, Fiber: 7 g

HEALTH BENEFITS:

Seasonal Produce Swap: Replace zucchini with sweet potatoes in winter.
Dietary Substitutions: Serve with whole-grain bread for a more filling meal.

BUDGET-FRIENDLY RECIPES

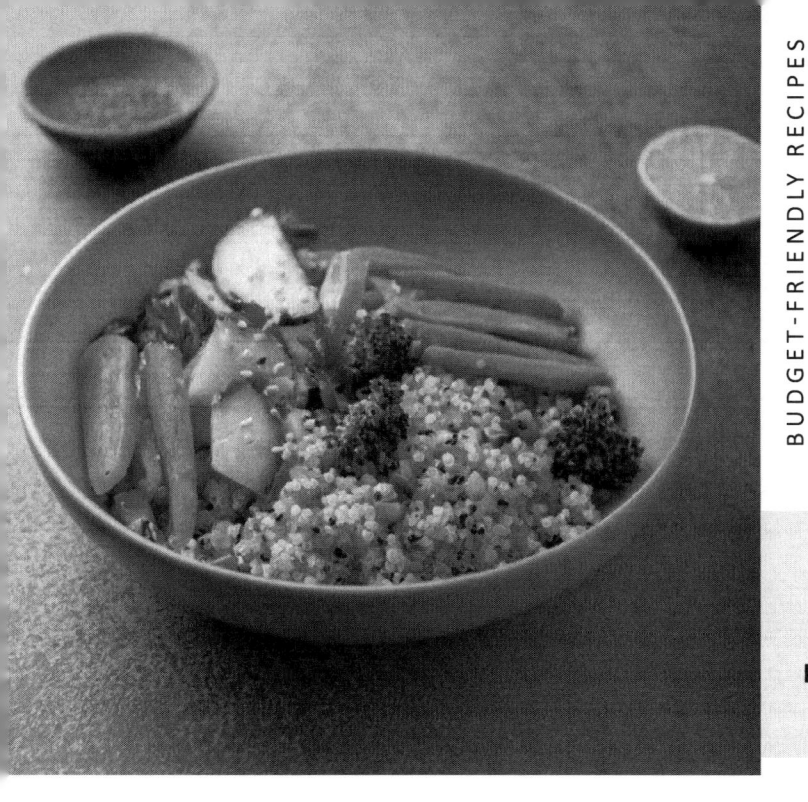

SIMPLE QUINOA AND VEGGIE BOWL

Anti-Inflammatory Benefits:
Quinoa is a complete protein and contains anti-inflammatory phytonutrients, while vegetables provide essential vitamins and antioxidants.

PREP TIME: 10 MINS
COOK TIME: 15 MINS
SERVING: 3 Portion Size: 1 bowl per serving

INGREDIENTS

- 1 cup (170 g) cooked quinoa
- 1/2 cup (50 g) broccoli florets
- 1/2 cup (50 g) diced zucchini
- 1/2 cup (50 g) diced red bell pepper
- 1 tbsp (15 ml) olive oil
- Salt and pepper to taste

INSTRUCTIONS

1. In a skillet, heat one tbsp oil over moderate stove flame. Add broccoli, zucchini, and bell pepper. Sauté for 5–7 minutes until tender.
2. Add preared quinoa and stir to combine.
3. Powder it with salt and crushed pepper, then serve warm.

EQUIPMENT NEEDED:
Saucepan, skillet

NUTRITIONAL INFORMATION (PER SERVING):

Calories: 180 kcal, Carbohydrates: 25 g, Protein: 6 g, Fat: 6 g, Fiber: 4 g

HEALTH BENEFITS:
Seasonal Produce Swap: Add asparagus or peas in spring.
Dietary Substitutions: Replace quinoa with brown rice or bulgur.

BUDGET-FRIENDLY RECIPES

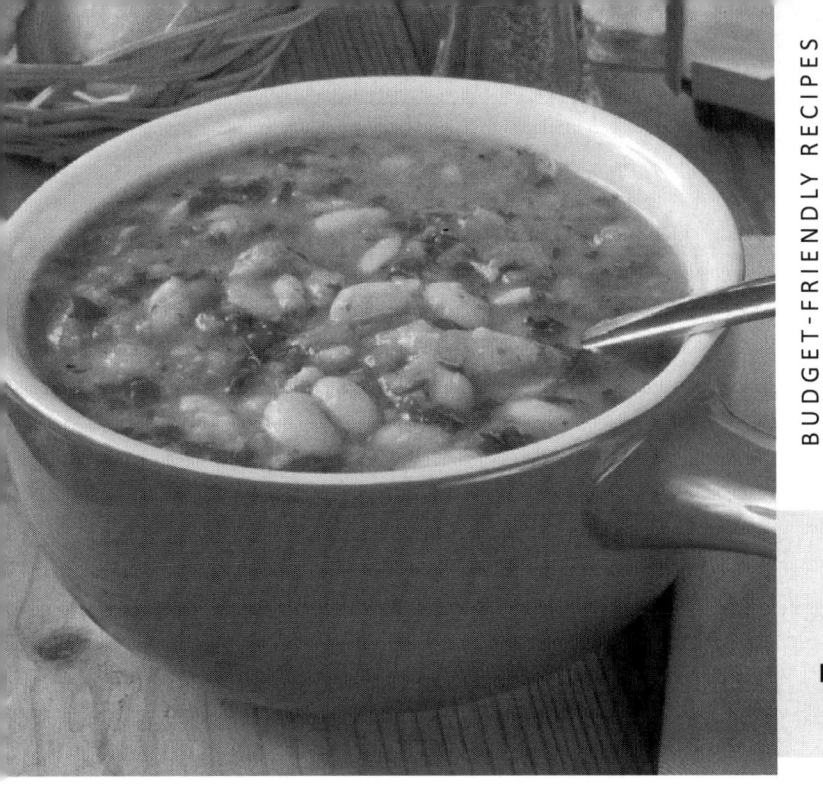

WHITE BEAN AND KALE SOUP

Anti-Inflammatory Benefits:
White beans are a good source of protein and fiber, while kale provides antioxidants and vitamin K, both of which combat inflammation.

PREP TIME: 10 MINS

COOK TIME: 20 MINS

SERVING: 4
Portion Size: 1 bowl per serving

INGREDIENTS

- 1 cup (150 g weight) canned white beans (drained and rinsed)
- 2 cups (60 g) chopped kale
- 1/2 cup (50 g) diced carrots
- 1/4 cup (30 g) diced onion
- 2 cups (480 ml) vegetable broth
- 1 tbsp (15 ml) olive oil
- Salt and pepper to taste

EQUIPMENT NEEDED:
Large pot, spoon

INSTRUCTIONS

1. Heat one tbsp oil in a pot over moderate stove flame. Add chopped onion and carrots, and sauté for 3 minutes.
2. Toss in the white beans and vegetable broth. Simmer for 10 minutes.
3. Add kale and cook more for another 5 minutes, until wilted.
4. Powder it with salt and crushed pepper, then serve warm.

NUTRITIONAL INFORMATION (PER SERVING):

Calories: 130 kcal, Carbohydrates: 20 g, Protein: 5 g, Fat: 4 g, Fiber: 6 g

HEALTH BENEFITS:

Seasonal Produce Swap: Use spinach or Swiss chard instead of kale.
Dietary Substitutions: Add quinoa for a heartier soup.

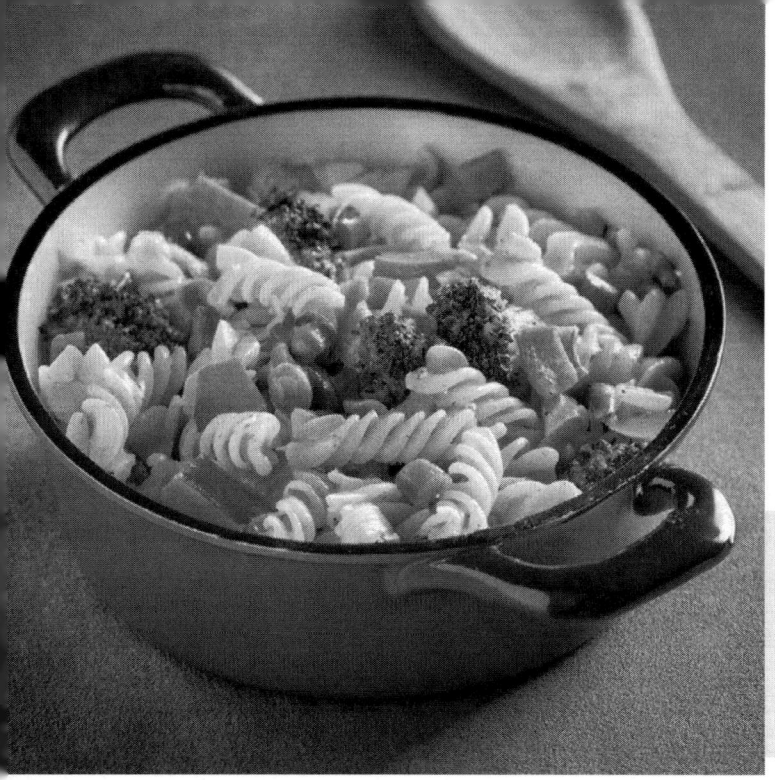

BUDGET-FRIENDLY RECIPES

ONE-POT PASTA WITH VEGGIES

Anti-Inflammatory Benefits:
Whole-grain pasta adds fiber to support gut health, while vegetables like zucchini and spinach provide essential anti-inflammatory nutrients.

PREP TIME: 10 MINS

COOK TIME: 20 MINS

SERVING: 4
Portion Size: 1 bowl per serving

INGREDIENTS

- 2 cups (200 g) whole-grain pasta
- 1 cup (100 g) diced zucchini
- 1 cup (30 g) fresh spinach
- 1/2 cup (75 g) cherry tomatoes, halved
- 2 cups (480 ml) vegetable broth
- 1 tbsp (15 ml) olive oil
- Salt and pepper to taste

INSTRUCTIONS

1. In a pot, combine the pasta, zucchini, cherry tomatoes, vegetable broth, and olive oil.
2. Get it to a boil, then decrease the stove heat and simmer for 15–20 minutes, keep stirring occasionally, until the pasta is done thoroughly and most of the liquid is absorbed.
3. Toss in the spinach during the last 2 minutes of cooking.
4. Powder it with salt and crushed pepper, then serve warm.

EQUIPMENT NEEDED:
Large pot, spoon

NUTRITIONAL INFORMATION (PER SERVING):

Calories: 200 kcal, Carbohydrates: 35 g, Protein: 6 g, Fat: 5 g, Fiber: 5 g

HEALTH BENEFITS:
Seasonal Produce Swap: Add asparagus or mushrooms in spring.
Dietary Substitutions: Use gluten-free pasta if needed.

BUDGET-FRIENDLY RECIPES

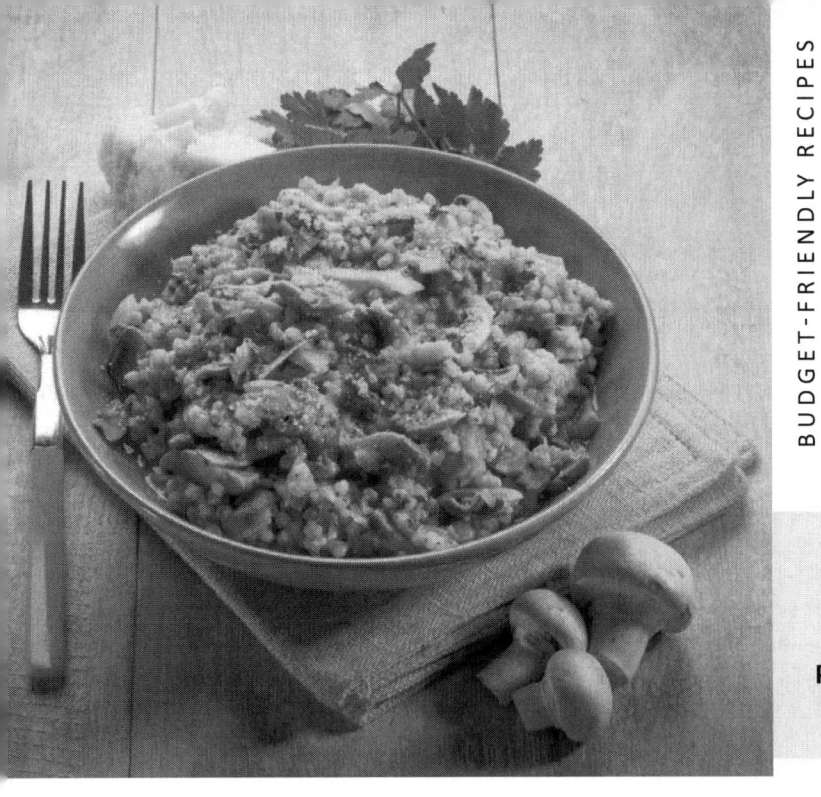

BARLEY AND MUSHROOM RISOTTO

Anti-Inflammatory Benefits:
Barley is rich in fiber, which supports gut health and reduces inflammation, while mushrooms contain antioxidants and anti-inflammatory compounds.

PREP TIME: 10 MINS

COOK TIME: 30 MINS

SERVING: 4
Portion Size: 1 bowl per serving

INGREDIENTS

- 1 cup (200 g) pearl barley
- 2 cups (480 ml) vegetable broth
- 1 cup (100 g) mushrooms, sliced
- 1/2 cup (50 g) diced onion
- 1 clove garlic, minced
- 1 tbsp (15 ml) olive oil
- Salt and pepper to taste

EQUIPMENT NEEDED:
Large skillet, saucepan, spoon

INSTRUCTIONS

1. Heat one tbsp oil in a skillet over moderate stove flame. Add chopped onion and garlic, and sauté for 3 minutes.
2. Add mushroom slices and softened for 5 minutes, until tender.
3. Toss in the barley and cook for 1 minute to toast lightly.
4. Gradually add vegetable broth, 1/2 cup at a time, stirring frequently until absorbed. Repeat until the barley is tender and creamy, about 25 minutes.
5. Powder it with salt and crushed pepper, then serve warm.

NUTRITIONAL INFORMATION (PER SERVING):

Calories: 180 kcal, Carbohydrates: 32 g, Protein: 5 g, Fat: 3 g, Fiber: 5 g

HEALTH BENEFITS:
Seasonal Produce Swap: Add spinach or kale for extra greens.
Dietary Substitutions: Use farro instead of barley for a different grain.

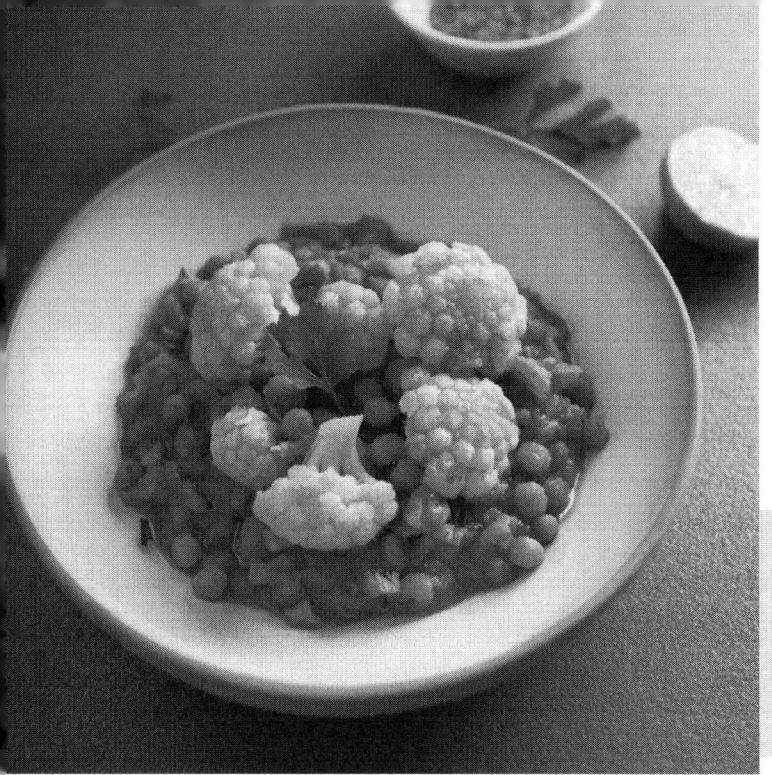

BUDGET-FRIENDLY RECIPES

CAULIFLOWER AND LENTIL CURRY

Anti-Inflammatory Benefits:
Cauliflower is a cruciferous vegetable rich in antioxidants, while lentils provide fiber and protein to support gut health and reduce inflammation.

PREP TIME: 10 MINS
COOK TIME: 25 MINS
SERVING: 3
Portion Size: 1 bowl per serving

INGREDIENTS

- 1 cup (150 g) cooked lentils
- 2 cups (200 g) cauliflower florets
- 1/2 cup (100 g) diced tomatoes
- 1/2 cup (120 ml) coconut milk
- 1/2 onion (50 g), diced
- 1 tsp (2 g) ground turmeric
- 1/2 tsp (1 g) ground cumin
- 1 tbsp (15 ml) olive oil

EQUIPMENT NEEDED:
Large pot, spoon

INSTRUCTIONS

1. Heat one tbsp oil in a pot over moderate stove flame. Add chopped onion and softened for 3 minutes.
2. Toss in the turmeric and cumin, and cook for 1 minute until fragrant.
3. Add tomatoes, lentils, and coconut milk. Simmer for 10 minutes.
4. Add cauliflower and cook for more 10 minutes, until tender.
5. Serve warm with fresh cilantro.

NUTRITIONAL INFORMATION (PER SERVING):

Calories: 220 kcal, Carbohydrates: 24 g, Protein: 8 g, Fat: 10 g, Fiber: 6 g

HEALTH BENEFITS:
Seasonal Produce Swap: Replace cauliflower with broccoli or sweet potato.
Dietary Substitutions: Use chickpeas instead of lentils for variety.

BUDGET-FRIENDLY RECIPES

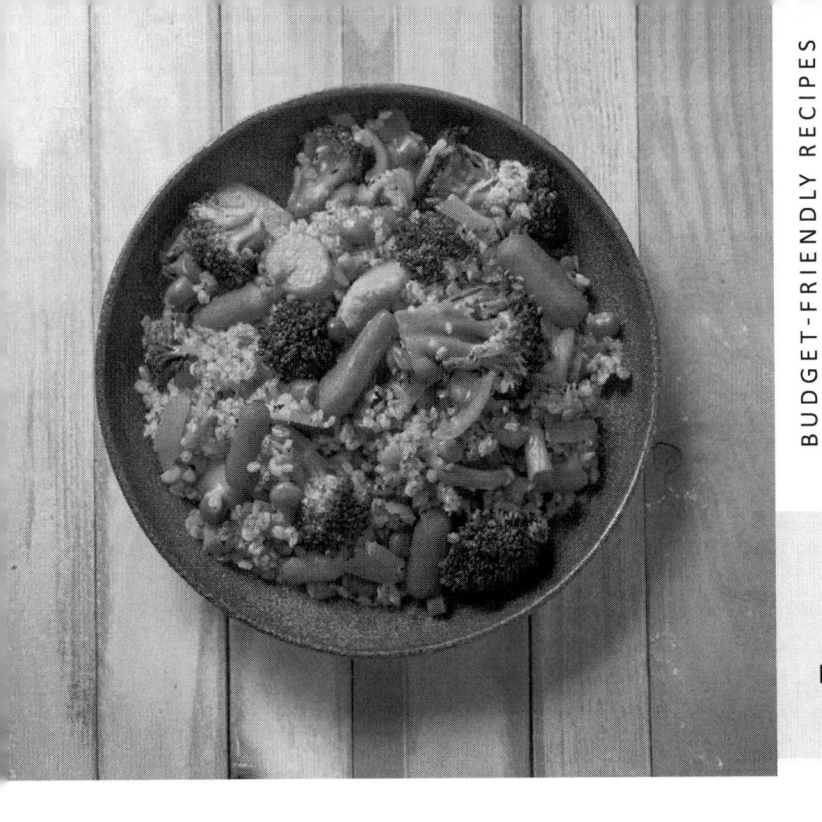

WHOLE WHEAT VEGETABLE STIR-FRY

Anti-Inflammatory Benefits:
Whole wheat noodles provide fiber to support gut health, while vegetables like bell peppers and broccoli are loaded with antioxidants and vitamins.

PREP TIME: 10 MINS
COOK TIME: 15 MINS
SERVING: 3 Portion Size: 1 bowl per serving

INGREDIENTS

- 200 g whole wheat noodles
- 1 cup (100 g) broccoli florets
- 1/2 cup (50 g) sliced red bell pepper
- 1/2 cup (50 g) sliced zucchini
- 1 tbsp (15 ml) soy sauce (low-sodium)
- 1 tbsp (15 ml) olive oil
- Salt and pepper to taste

INSTRUCTIONS

1. Cook the whole wheat noodles according to the mentioned steps on the the package instructions. Drain and set aside.
2. Heat one tbsp oil in a skillet or wok over moderate stove flame. Add broccoli, bell pepper, and zucchini, and stir-fry for 5–7 minutes.
3. Add cooked noodles and soy sauce, tossing to combine. Cook for another 2 minutes.
4. Powder it with salt and crushed pepper, then serve immediately.

NUTRITIONAL INFORMATION (PER SERVING):

Calories: 220 kcal, Carbohydrates: 40 g, Protein: 6 g, Fat: 5 g, Fiber: 6 g

HEALTH BENEFITS:
Seasonal Produce Swap: Add asparagus or snap peas in spring.
Dietary Substitutions: Use rice noodles as a gluten-free option.

EQUIPMENT NEEDED:
Skillet or wok, saucepan, spatula

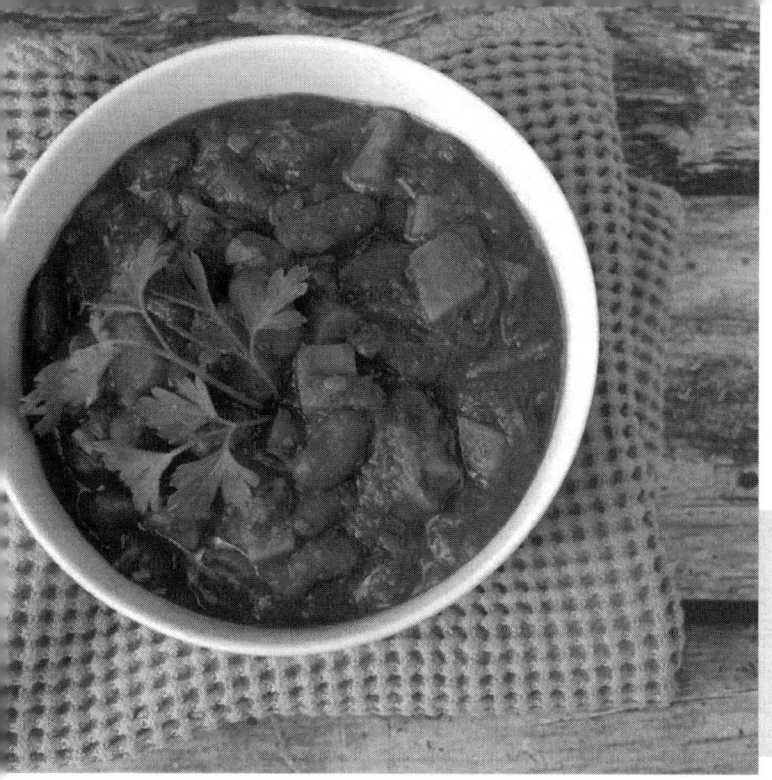

BUDGET-FRIENDLY RECIPES

SWEET POTATO AND BLACK BEAN CHILI

Anti-Inflammatory Benefits:
Sweet potatoes are rich in beta-carotene, while black beans provide protein and fiber, making this chili hearty and anti-inflammatory.

PREP TIME: 10 MINS

COOK TIME: 25 MINS

SERVING: 4
Portion Size: 1 bowl per serving

INGREDIENTS

- 1 medium sweet potato (150 g), diced
- 1 cup (150 g) black beans (cooked or canned, drained and rinsed)
- 1/2 cup (75 g) diced tomatoes
- 1/2 cup (50 g) diced onion
- 2 cups (480 ml) vegetable broth
- 1 tsp (2 g) ground cumin
- 1/2 tsp (1 g) chili powder

EQUIPMENT NEEDED:
Large pot, spoon

INSTRUCTIONS

1. Heat a small amount of oil in a pot over a moderate stove flame. Add chopped onion and sweet potato and cook for 5 minutes.
2. Toss in cumin and chili powder and cook for 1 minute until fragrant.
3. Add black beans, tomatoes, and vegetable broth. Get it to a boil, then decrease the stove heat and simmer for 20 minutes.
4. Serve warm with optional toppings like fresh cilantro or avocado slices.

NUTRITIONAL INFORMATION (PER SERVING):

Calories: 190 kcal, Carbohydrates: 32 g, Protein: 6 g, Fat: 2 g, Fiber: 7 g

HEALTH BENEFITS:

Seasonal Produce Swap: Add corn or zucchini in summer for extra flavor. **Dietary Substitutions:** Serve with whole-grain bread for a heartier meal.

SEASONAL PRODUCE RECIPES

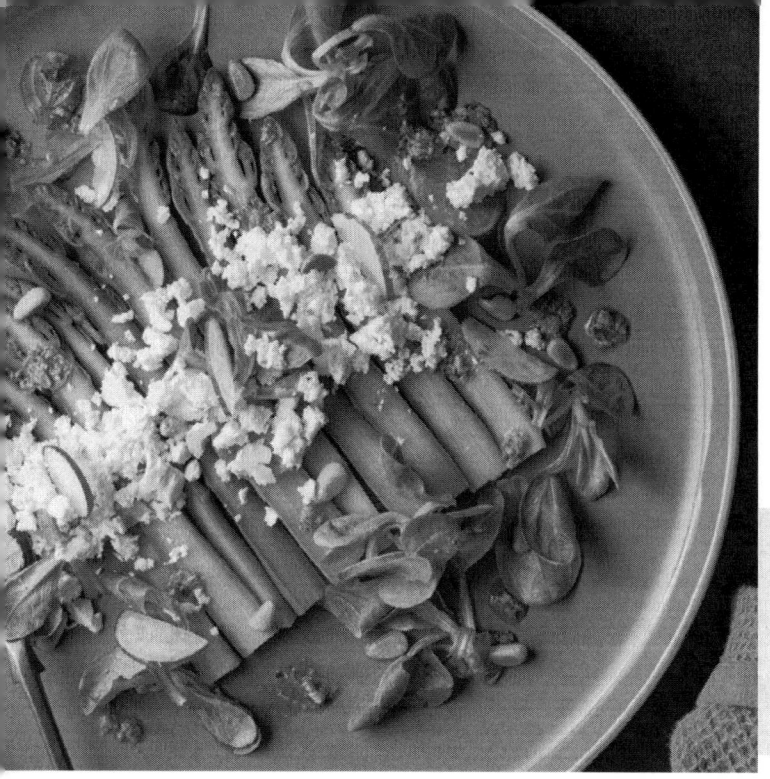

SEASONAL PRODUCE RECIPES

SPRING ASPARAGUS AND SPINACH SALAD

Anti-Inflammatory Benefits:
Asparagus is high in antioxidants and anti-inflammatory nutrients, while spinach provides a rich source of vitamins and minerals to combat inflammation.

PREP TIME: 10 MINS
COOK TIME: 00 MINS
SERVING: 2
Portion Size: 1 bowl per serving

INGREDIENTS

- 1 cup (150 g) fresh asparagus, trimmed and sliced
- 2 cups (60 g) fresh spinach leaves
- 1/4 cup (40 g) cherry tomatoes, halved
- 2 tbsp (30 ml) olive oil
- 1 tbsp (15 ml) lemon juice
- Salt and pepper to taste

EQUIPMENT NEEDED:
Knife, mixing bowl

INSTRUCTIONS

1. In a large, deep-bottom bowl, combine the asparagus, spinach, and cherry tomatoes.
2. Drizzle two tbsp oil and lemon juice, then powder it with salt and crushed pepper.
3. Toss gently and serve immediately.

NUTRITIONAL INFORMATION (PER SERVING):

Calories: 120 kcal, Carbohydrates: 5 g, Protein: 3 g, Fat: 10 g, Fiber: 3 g

HEALTH BENEFITS:
Seasonal Produce Swap: Add radishes or peas for extra crunch.
Dietary Substitutions: Add a sprinkle of feta cheese for a richer flavor.

SEASONAL PRODUCE RECIPES

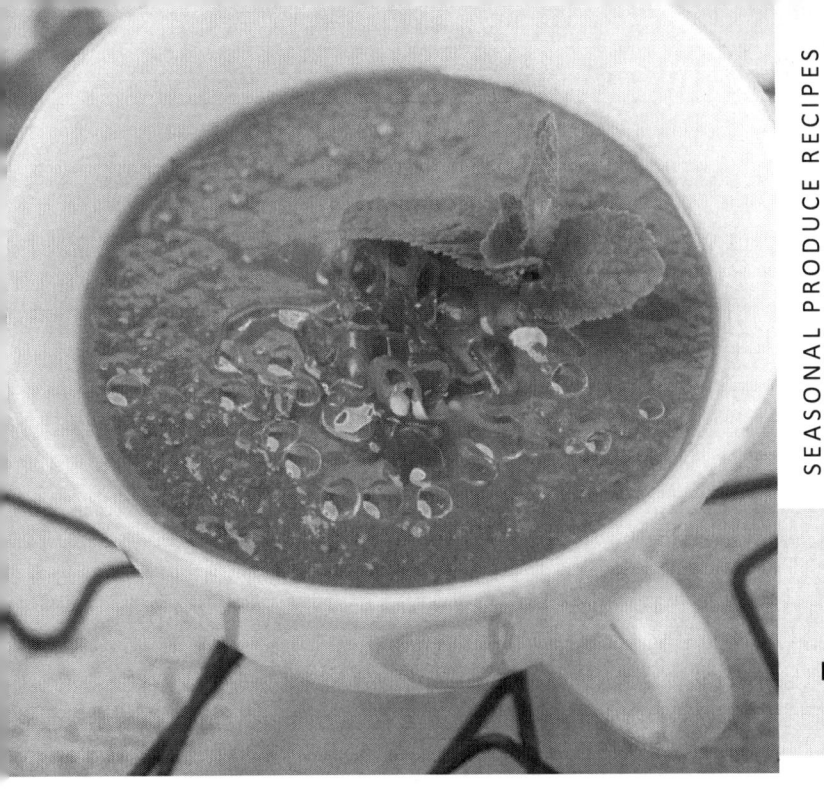

SUMMER TOMATO AND BASIL GAZPACHO

Anti-Inflammatory Benefits:
Tomatoes are rich in lycopene, an antioxidant that reduces inflammation, and fresh basil provides anti-inflammatory essential oils.

PREP TIME: 15 MINS

COOK TIME: 00 MINS

SERVING: 3
Portion Size: 1 bowl per serving

INGREDIENTS

- 3 large tomatoes (450 g), chopped
- 1/2 cucumber (75 g), peeled and diced
- 1 red bell pepper (100 g), diced
- 1/4 cup (30 g) diced onion
- 2 tbsp (30 ml) olive oil
- 1 tbsp (15 ml) red wine vinegar
- 1/4 cup (10 g) basil leaves

EQUIPMENT NEEDED:
Blender or food processor, knife

INSTRUCTIONS

1. In a food blender, combine the tomatoes, cucumber, bell pepper, onion, olive oil, and red wine vinegar. Blend on full power until the ingredient's texture looks smooth.
2. Toss in the basil leaves and refrigerate for at least 1 hour.
3. Serve chilled, and spread additional basil on top if desired.

NUTRITIONAL INFORMATION (PER SERVING):

Calories: 130 kcal, Carbohydrates: 12 g, Protein: 2 g, Fat: 9 g, Fiber: 3 g

HEALTH BENEFITS:
Seasonal Produce Swap: Add fresh corn or zucchini for a summer twist.
Dietary Substitutions: Use apple cider vinegar instead of red wine vinegar for a different flavor.

SEASONAL PRODUCE RECIPES

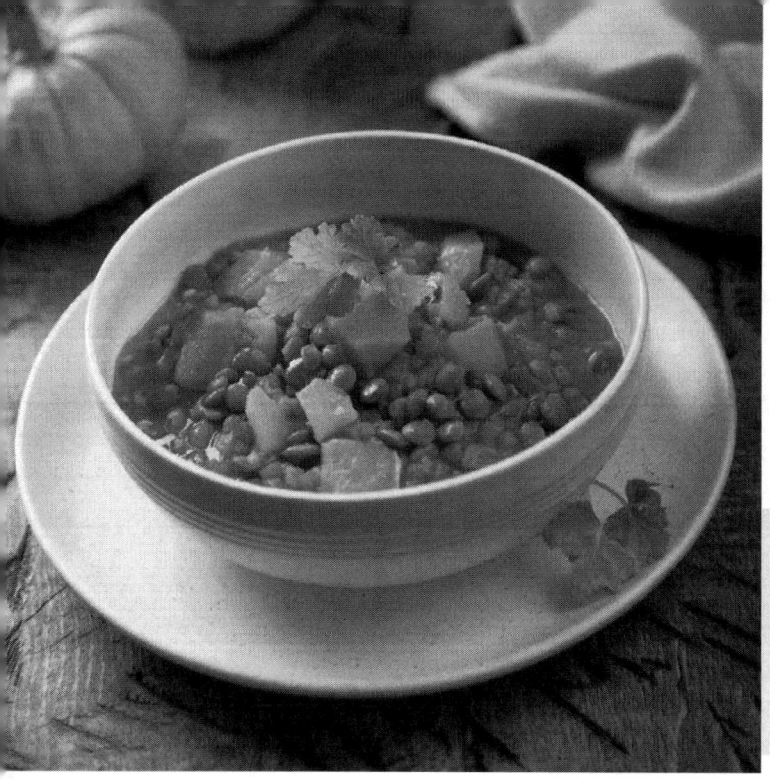

AUTUMN PUMPKIN AND LENTIL STEW

Anti-Inflammatory Benefits:
Pumpkin is rich in beta-carotene, an anti-inflammatory antioxidant, while lentils provide fiber and plant-based protein to support gut health.

PREP TIME: 10 MINS

COOK TIME: 25 MINS

SERVING: 3
Portion Size: 1 bowl per serving

INGREDIENTS

- 1 cup (150 g) cooked lentils
- 1 cup (200 g) diced pumpkin
- 1/2 cup (100 g) diced tomatoes
- 1/2 onion (50 g), diced
- 2 cups (480 ml) vegetable broth
- 1/2 tsp (1 g) ground cinnamon
- 1 tbsp (15 ml) olive oil

EQUIPMENT NEEDED:
Pot, spoon

INSTRUCTIONS

1. Heat one tbsp oil in a pot over moderate stove flame. Add chopped onion and softened for 3 minutes.
2. Toss in the pumpkin, tomatoes, and cinnamon. Cook for 5 minutes.
3. Add lentils and vegetable broth, and get it to a simmer. Cook for 17–20 minutes until the pumpkin gets tender.
4. Serve warm with fresh parsley on top.

NUTRITIONAL INFORMATION (PER SERVING):

Calories: 180 kcal, Carbohydrates: 26 g, Protein: 7 g, Fat: 4 g, Fiber: 8 g

HEALTH BENEFITS:

Seasonal Produce Swap: Use butternut squash or sweet potatoes instead of pumpkin.
Dietary Substitutions: Add coconut milk for a creamier stew.

SEASONAL PRODUCE RECIPES

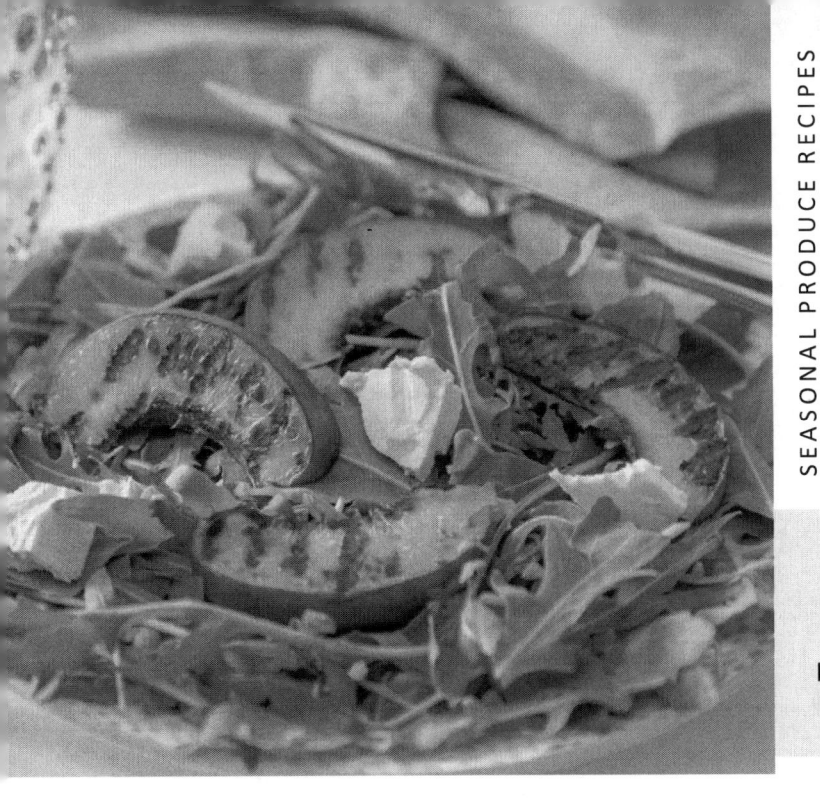

SUMMER GRILLED PEACH SALAD

Anti-Inflammatory Benefits:
Peaches are high in antioxidants and vitamin C, while spinach adds anti-inflammatory nutrients like vitamin K and magnesium.

PREP TIME: 10 MINS

COOK TIME: 5 MINS

SERVING: 2
Portion Size: 1 bowl per serving

INGREDIENTS

- 2 fresh peaches (200 g), halved and pitted
- 2 cups (60 g) fresh spinach leaves
- 1/4 cup (40 g) crumbled goat cheese
- 2 tbsp (30 ml) balsamic glaze

EQUIPMENT NEEDED:
Grill pan, knife, mixing bowl

INSTRUCTIONS

1. Preheat grill pan over moderate stove flame. Grill the peach halves for 2–3 minutes on one side until lightly charred.
2. Take a large, deep-bottom bowl and combine the spinach and grilled peaches.
3. Top with crumbled goat cheese, then drizzle balsamic glaze.
4. Serve immediately.

NUTRITIONAL INFORMATION (PER SERVING):

Calories: 150 kcal, Carbohydrates: 12 g, Protein: 4 g, Fat: 8 g, Fiber: 3 g

HEALTH BENEFITS:
Seasonal Produce Swap: Substitute peaches with nectarines or plums.
Dietary Substitutions: Use dairy-free cheese for a vegan option.

SEASONAL PRODUCE RECIPES

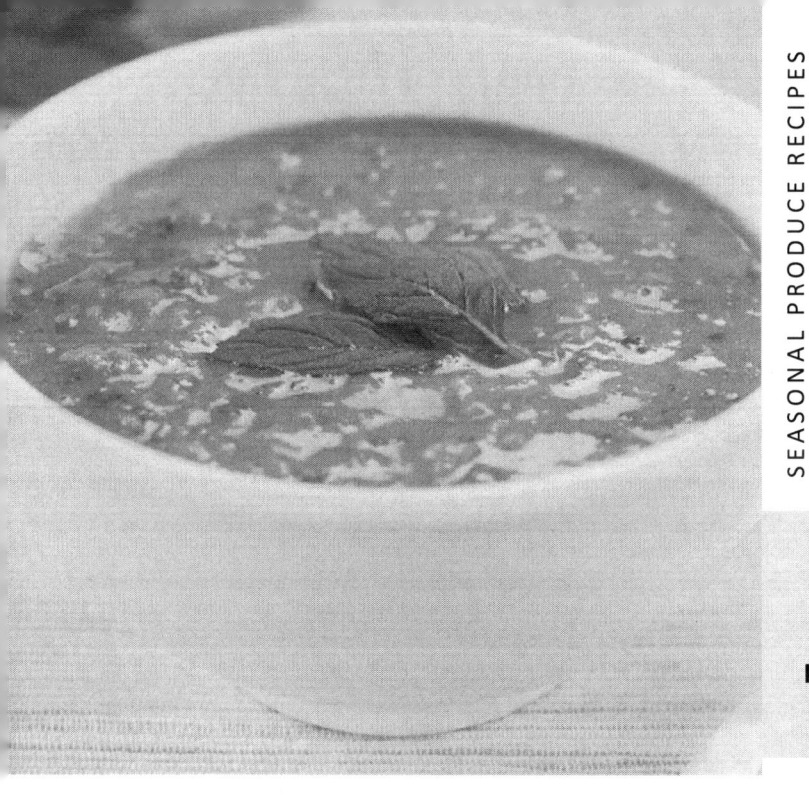

SPRING PEA AND MINT SOUP

Anti-Inflammatory Benefits:
Peas are a great source of plant-based protein and fiber, while mint has anti-inflammatory and soothing properties.

PREP TIME: 10 MINS

COOK TIME: 15 MINS

SERVING: 3
Portion Size: 1 bowl per serving

INGREDIENTS

- 2 cups (300 g) fresh peas
- 1/2 onion (50 g), diced
- 2 cups (480 ml) vegetable broth
- 1/4 cup (10 g) mint leaves
- 1 tbsp (15 ml) olive oil
- Salt and pepper to taste

EQUIPMENT NEEDED:
Pot, blender

INSTRUCTIONS

1. Heat one tbsp oil in a pot over moderate stove flame. Add chopped onion and softened for 3 minutes.
2. Toss in the peas and vegetable broth. Simmer for 10 minutes.
3. Remove from heat and blend on full power until the ingredient's texture looks smooth.
4. Toss in the mint leaves, powder it with salt and crushed pepper, and serve warm or chilled.

NUTRITIONAL INFORMATION (PER SERVING):

Calories: 120 kcal, Carbohydrates: 18 g, Protein: 5 g, Fat: 4 g, Fiber: 4 g

HEALTH BENEFITS:
Seasonal Produce Swap: Add asparagus or zucchini in spring for extra flavor.
Dietary Substitutions: Use coconut milk for a creamier texture.

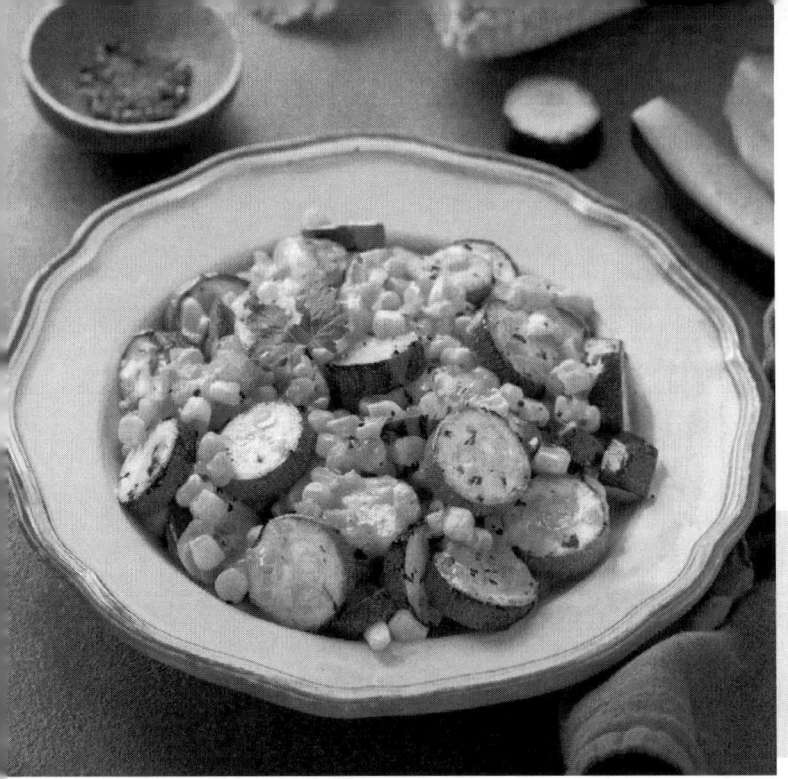

SEASONAL PRODUCE RECIPES

SUMMER CORN AND ZUCCHINI SAUTÉ

Anti-Inflammatory Benefits:
Corn provides fiber and essential vitamins, while zucchini is low in calories and rich in antioxidants that help reduce inflammation.

PREP TIME: 10 MINS

COOK TIME: 10 MINS

SERVING: 3
Portion Size: 1 bowl per serving

INGREDIENTS

- 1 cup (150 g) fresh corn kernels (from 1–2 ears of corn)
- 1 medium zucchini (150 g), diced
- 1/2 red bell pepper (50 g), diced
- 1 clove garlic, minced
- 1 tbsp (15 ml) olive oil
- Salt and pepper to taste

EQUIPMENT NEEDED:
Skillet, knife, spatula

INSTRUCTIONS

1. Heat one tbsp oil in a skillet over moderate stove flame. Add garlic and sauté for 1 minute until fragrant.
2. Add corn, zucchini, and bell pepper. Cook for 5–7 minutes, keep stirring occasionally, until the vegetables are tender but still crisp.
3. Powder it with salt and crushed pepper, and serve immediately.

NUTRITIONAL INFORMATION (PER SERVING):

Calories: 120 kcal, Carbohydrates: 20 g, Protein: 3 g, Fat: 4 g, Fiber: 3 g

HEALTH BENEFITS:
Seasonal Produce Swap: Add cherry tomatoes or fresh basil for a summer twist.
Dietary Substitutions: Use ghee instead of olive oil for a buttery flavor.

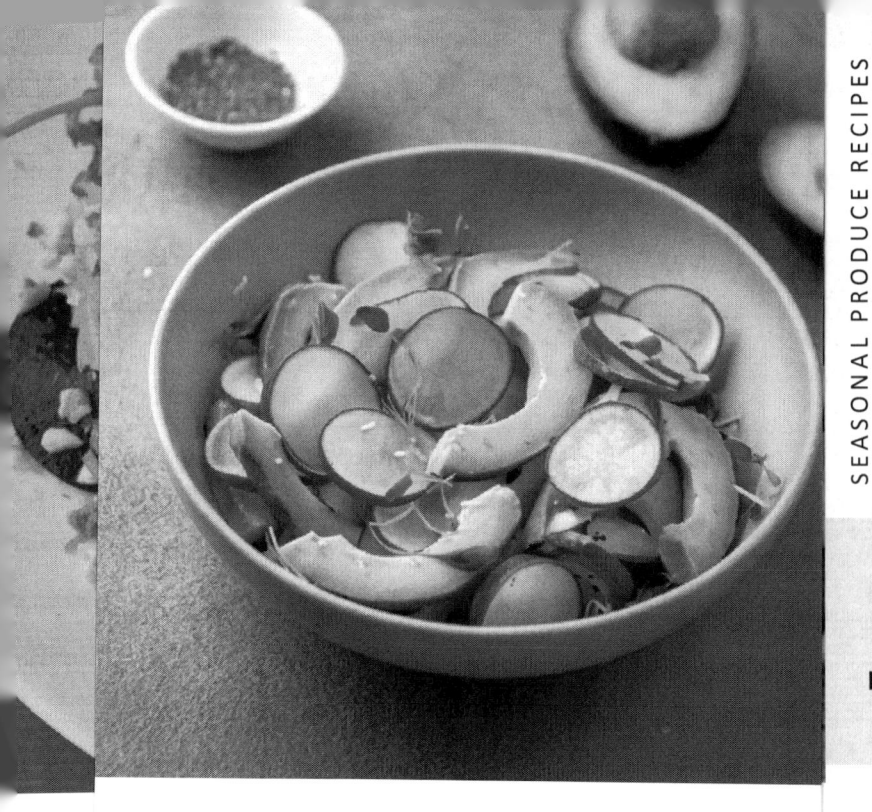

WINTER CARROT AND PARSNIP ROAST

SEASONAL PRODUCE RECIPES

Anti-Inflammatory Benefits:
Carrots and parsnips are rich in antioxidants like beta-carotene and vitamin C, which support immune health and reduce inflammation.

PREP TIME: 10 MINS
COOK TIME: 30 MINS
SERVING: 3
Portion Size: 1 bowl per serving

INGREDIENTS

- 1 cup (100 g) radishes, thinly sliced
- 1 avocado (150 g), diced
- 2 cups (60 g) mixed greens
- 1 tbsp (15 ml) lemon juice
- 1 tbsp (15 ml) olive oil
- Salt and pepper to taste

EQUIPMENT NEEDED:
Knife, mixing bowl

INSTRUCTIONS

1. Take oven to 400°F (200°C). and e carrots and parsnips on the paper-arranged baking sheet.
2. Drizzne tbsp oil, sprinkle with thyme, and powder it with salt and cruspepper. Toss to coat evenly.
3. Toss 25–30 minutes, stirring after the halftime has passed until the es are tender and golden.
   rm.

NRITIONAL INFORMATION (PER SERVING):

Calories:) kcal, Carbohydrates: 22 g, Protein: 2 g, Fat: 4 g, Fiber: 6 g

HEALTH NEFITS:
Seasonaoduce Swap: Add turnips or Brussels sprouts for variety.
radishes. **stitutions:** Use coconut oil instead of olive oil for a different
Dietary

69

SUPERFOODS RECIPES

SUPERFOODS RECIPES

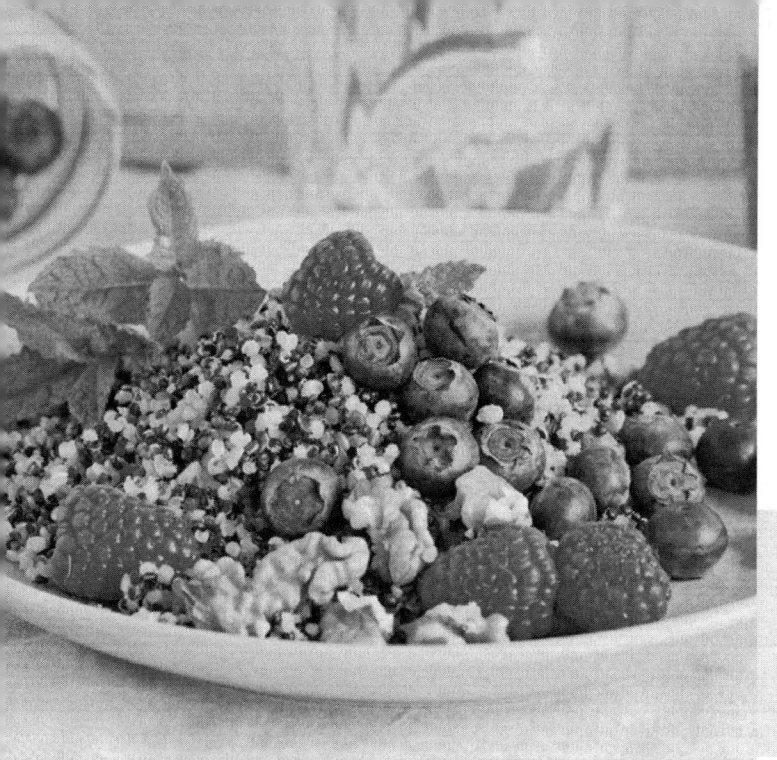

QUINOA SALAD WITH BLUEBERRIES AND WALNUTS

Anti-Inflammatory Benefits:
Quinoa is a complete protein with anti-inflammatory phytonutrients, blueberries are rich in antioxidants, and walnuts provide omega-3 fatty acids.

PREP TIME: 10 MINS

COOK TIME: 15 MINS

SERVING: 2
Portion Size: 1 bowl per serving

INGREDIENTS

- 1/2 cup (90 g) quinoa, rinsed
- 1 cup (240 ml) water
- 1/2 cup (75 g) fresh blueberries
- 1/4 cup (30 g) walnuts, chopped
- 2 tbsp (30 ml) olive oil
- 1 tbsp (15 ml) lemon juice
- Salt and pepper to taste

EQUIPMENT NEEDED:
Saucepan, mixing bowl

INSTRUCTIONS

1. Combine the quinoa with water in a saucepan. Get it to a boil, then decrease the stove heat and simmer for 15 minutes or until the quinoa is tender and the water is absorbed. Let cool.
2. Take a large, deep-bottom bowl and combine the quinoa, blueberries, and walnuts.
3. Drizzle two tbsp oil and lemon juice, powder it with salt and crushed pepper, and toss to combine.
4. Serve immediately.

NUTRITIONAL INFORMATION (PER SERVING):

Calories: 220 kcal, Carbohydrates: 22 g, Protein: 6 g, Fat: 12 g, Fiber: 4 g

HEALTH BENEFITS:
Seasonal Produce Swap: Substitute blueberries with strawberries or pomegranate seeds.
Dietary Substitutions: Add crumbled goat cheese for a richer flavor.

SUPERFOODS RECIPES

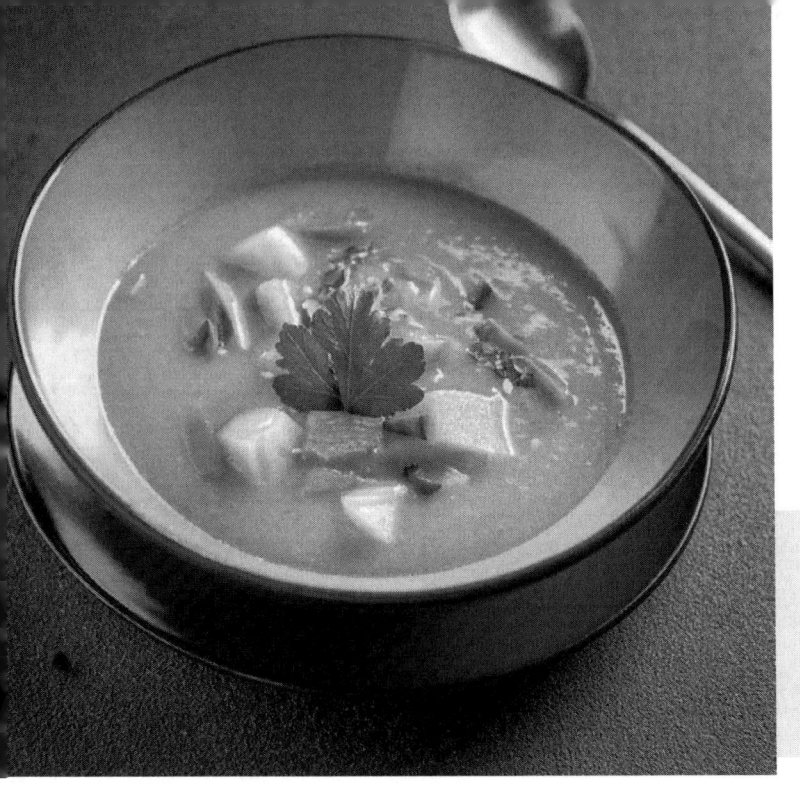

TURMERIC AND GINGER VEGETABLE SOUP

Anti-Inflammatory Benefits:
Turmeric and ginger are powerful anti-inflammatory spices, while vegetables provide essential antioxidants and vitamins.

PREP TIME: 10 MINS

COOK TIME: 20 MINS

SERVING: 3
Portion Size: 1 bowl per serving

INGREDIENTS

- 1 cup (100 g) diced carrots
- 1/2 cup (50 g) diced celery
- 1/2 cup (50 g) diced onion
- 2 cups (480 ml) vegetable broth
- 1/2 tsp (1 g) ground turmeric
- 1/2 tsp (1 g) grated ginger
- 1 tbsp (15 ml) olive oil
- Salt and pepper to taste

INSTRUCTIONS

1. Heat one tbsp oil in a pot over moderate stove flame. Add chopped onion, carrots, and celery, and sauté for 5 minutes.
2. Toss in the turmeric and ginger, and cook for 1 minute.
3. Add vegetable broth and get it to a boil. Decrease the stove heat and simmer for 15 minutes until the vegetables are tender.
4. Powder it with salt and crushed pepper, then serve warm.

EQUIPMENT NEEDED:
Pot, spoon

NUTRITIONAL INFORMATION (PER SERVING):

Calories: 110 kcal, Carbohydrates: 12 g, Protein: 2 g, Fat: 6 g, Fiber: 3 g

HEALTH BENEFITS:
Seasonal Produce Swap: Add zucchini or spinach for extra greens.
Dietary Substitutions: Use chicken broth for added protein.

SUPERFOODS RECIPES

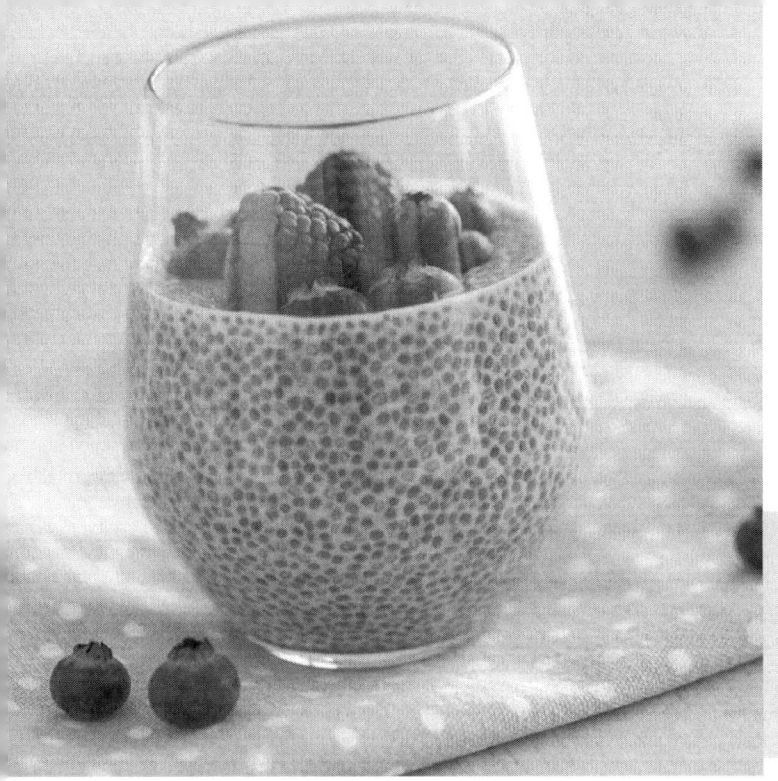

CHIA SEED PUDDING WITH RASPBERRIES

Anti-Inflammatory Benefits:
Chia seeds are rich in omega-3 fatty acids, while raspberries are packed with antioxidants to combat inflammation.

PREP TIME: 5 MINS

COOK TIME: 00 MINS

SERVING: 2
Portion Size: 1 bowl per serving

INGREDIENTS

- 1/4 cup (40 g) chia seeds
- 1 cup (240 ml) almond milk
- 1 tsp (5 ml) honey or maple syrup (optional)
- 1/2 cup (75 g) fresh raspberries

INSTRUCTIONS

1. Take a large, deep-bottom bowl and combine chia seeds, almond milk, and honey (if using). Stir well.
2. Cover and refrigerate for 4 hours (at least) or 6-8 hours until thickened.
3. Before serving, stir again and top with fresh raspberries.

EQUIPMENT NEEDED:
Mixing bowl, spoon

NUTRITIONAL INFORMATION (PER SERVING):

Calories: 150 kcal, Carbohydrates: 12 g, Protein: 5 g, Fat: 8 g, Fiber: 7 g

HEALTH BENEFITS:
Seasonal Produce Swap: Use strawberries, blueberries, or diced mango instead of raspberries.
Dietary Substitutions: Replace almond milk with oat milk for a nut-free option.

SUPERFOODS RECIPES

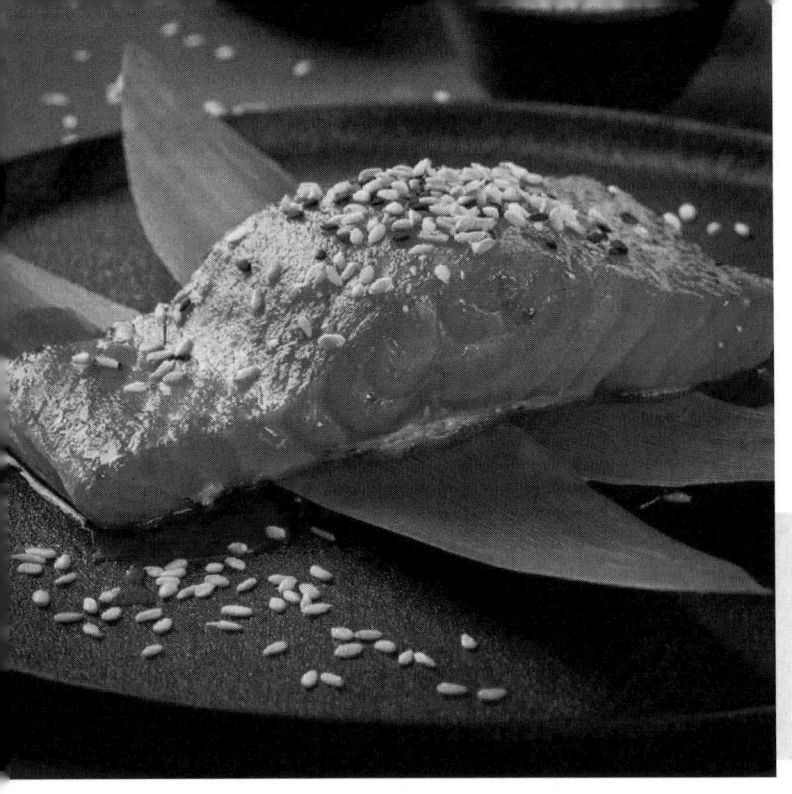

WILD SALMON WITH GINGER AND SESAME

Anti-Inflammatory Benefits:
Salmon is high in omega-3 fatty acids, which reduce inflammation, while ginger and sesame provide additional anti-inflammatory and antioxidant benefits.

PREP TIME: 10 MINS

COOK TIME: 15 MINS

SERVING: 2
Portion Size: 1 fillet per serving

INGREDIENTS

- 2 salmon fillets (300 g total)
- 1 tsp (5 ml) grated ginger
- 1 tbsp (15 ml) soy sauce (low-sodium)
- 1 tsp (5 ml) sesame oil
- 1 tbsp (15 g) sesame seeds

EQUIPMENT NEEDED:
Baking sheet, aluminum foil

INSTRUCTIONS

1. Preheat oven to 375°F (190°C).
2. Place the salmon fillets on the paper-arranged baking sheet lined with aluminum foil.
3. In a small bowl, combine grated ginger, soy sauce, and sesame oil. Brush the mixture over the salmon fillets.
4. Sprinkle sesame seeds on top.
5. Bake for 12–15 minutes until the fillet flakes easily. Serve warm.

NUTRITIONAL INFORMATION (PER SERVING):

Calories: 250 kcal, Carbohydrates: 2 g, Protein: 30 g, Fat: 12 g, Fiber: 1 g

HEALTH BENEFITS:
Seasonal Produce Swap: Serve with steamed asparagus or roasted Brussels sprouts.
Dietary Substitutions: Replace salmon with tofu or tempeh for a plant-based option.

SUPERFOODS RECIPES

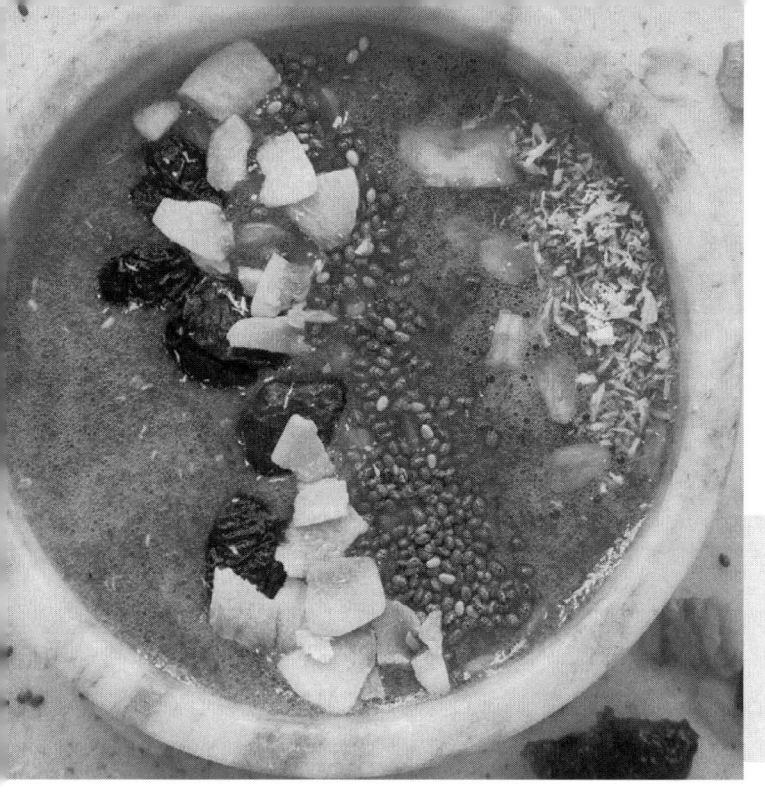

MATCHA GREEN SMOOTHIE BOWL

Anti-Inflammatory Benefits:
Matcha is rich in antioxidants like EGCG, which help reduce inflammation, while toppings like chia seeds and berries provide additional anti-inflammatory nutrients.

PREP TIME: 10 MINS

COOK TIME: 00 MINS

SERVING: 1
Portion Size: 1 bowl

INGREDIENTS

- 1/2 frozen banana (50 g)
- 1/2 cup (120 ml) almond milk
- 1 tsp (2 g) matcha green tea powder
- 1/4 cup (60 ml) Greek yogurt (optional)
- 1/4 cup (40 g) fresh berries (for topping)
- 1 tsp (5 g) chia seeds (for topping)

INSTRUCTIONS

1. In a food blender, combine frozen banana, almond milk, matcha powder, and Greek yogurt (if using). Blend on full power until the ingredient's texture looks smooth.
2. Pour into a wide-mouth bowl and top with fresh berries and chia seeds.
3. Serve immediately.

EQUIPMENT NEEDED:
Blender, bowl

NUTRITIONAL INFORMATION (PER SERVING):

Calories: 180 kcal, Carbohydrates: 20 g, Protein: 6 g, Fat: 7 g, Fiber: 5 g

HEALTH BENEFITS:
Seasonal Produce Swap: Use mango or kiwi instead of berries.
Dietary Substitutions: Replace Greek yogurt with coconut yogurt for a vegan option.

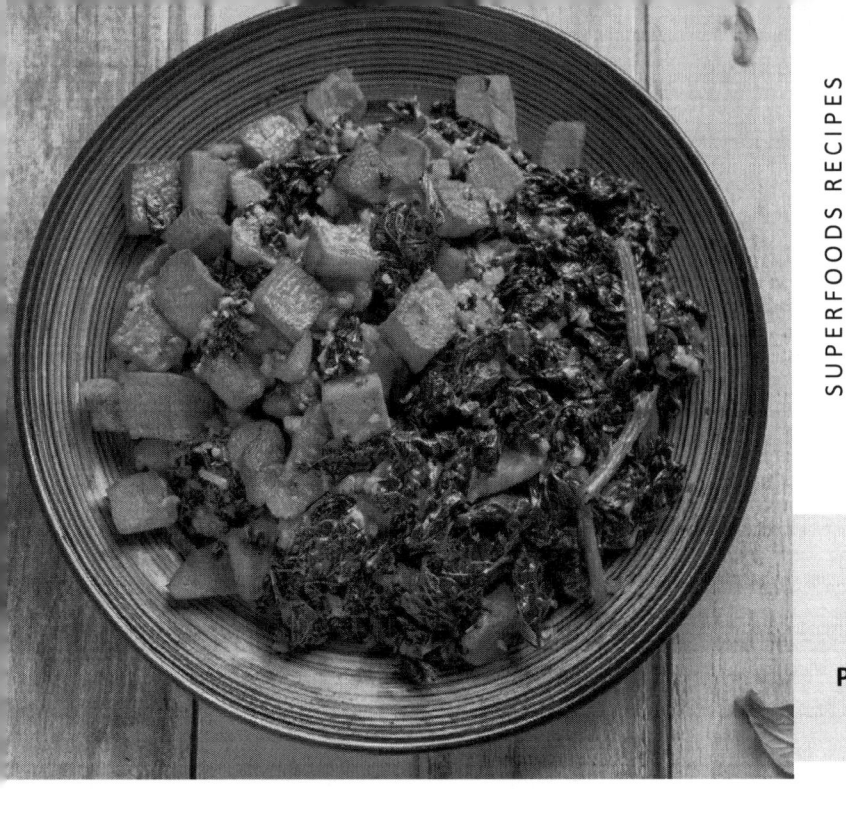

SPINACH AND SWEET POTATO HASH

SUPERFOODS RECIPES

Anti-Inflammatory Benefits:
Sweet potatoes are rich in beta-carotene, while spinach provides vitamins and antioxidants that support immune health and reduce inflammation.

PREP TIME: 10 MINS
COOK TIME: 15 MINS
SERVING: 2
Portion Size: 1 bowl per serving

INGREDIENTS

- 1 medium sweet potato (150 g), diced
- 1 cup (30 g) fresh spinach
- 1/2 small onion (25 g), diced
- 1 tbsp (15 ml) olive oil
- Salt and pepper to taste

EQUIPMENT NEEDED:
Skillet, knife, spatula

INSTRUCTIONS

1. Heat one tbsp oil in a skillet over moderate stove flame. Add diced sweet potato and onion, and sauté for 10 minutes, stirring occasionally.
2. Add spinach and cook for more 3–5 minutes until wilted.
3. Powder it with salt and crushed pepper, then serve immediately.

NUTRITIONAL INFORMATION (PER SERVING):
Calories: 180 kcal, Carbohydrates: 25 g, Protein: 3 g, Fat: 7 g, Fiber: 5 g

HEALTH BENEFITS:
Seasonal Produce Swap: Use kale or Swiss chard instead of spinach.
Dietary Substitutions: Add an egg on top for extra protein.

SUPERFOODS RECIPES

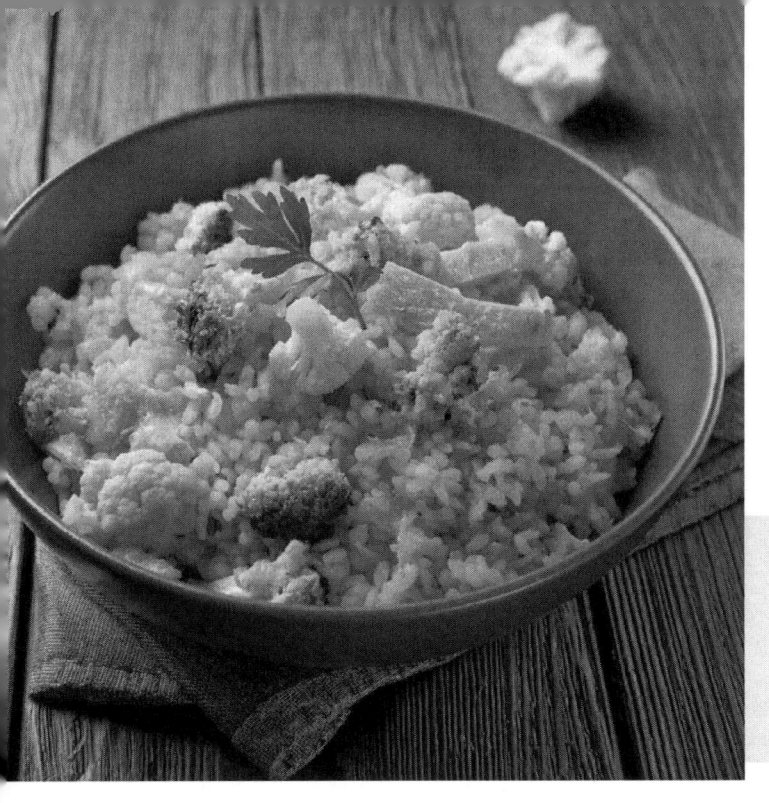

TURMERIC AND CAULIFLOWER RICE BOWL

Anti-Inflammatory Benefits:
Turmeric contains curcumin, a powerful anti-inflammatory compound, while cauliflower is packed with antioxidants.

PREP TIME: 10 MINS

COOK TIME: 10 MINS

SERVING: 2 Portion Size: 1 bowl per serving

INGREDIENTS

- 2 cups (200 g) cauliflower rice
- 1/2 cup (50 g) cooked chickpeas
- 1/4 cup (40 g) diced red bell pepper
- 1/2 tsp (1 g) ground turmeric
- 1 tbsp (15 ml) olive oil
- Salt and pepper to taste

INSTRUCTIONS

1. Heat one tbsp oil in a skillet over moderate stove flame. Add cauliflower rice and turmeric, and cook for 5–7 minutes, stirring occasionally.
2. Toss in the chickpeas and red bell pepper and cook for another 3 minutes.
3. Powder it with salt and crushed pepper, then serve warm.

NUTRITIONAL INFORMATION (PER SERVING):

Calories: 150 kcal, Carbohydrates: 12 g, Protein: 4 g, Fat: 8 g, Fiber: 4 g

HEALTH BENEFITS:

Seasonal Produce Swap: Add fresh peas or asparagus for a springtime twist.
Dietary Substitutions: Replace chickpeas with tofu for a different protein source.

EQUIPMENT NEEDED:
Skillet, knife, spatula

SUPERFOODS RECIPES

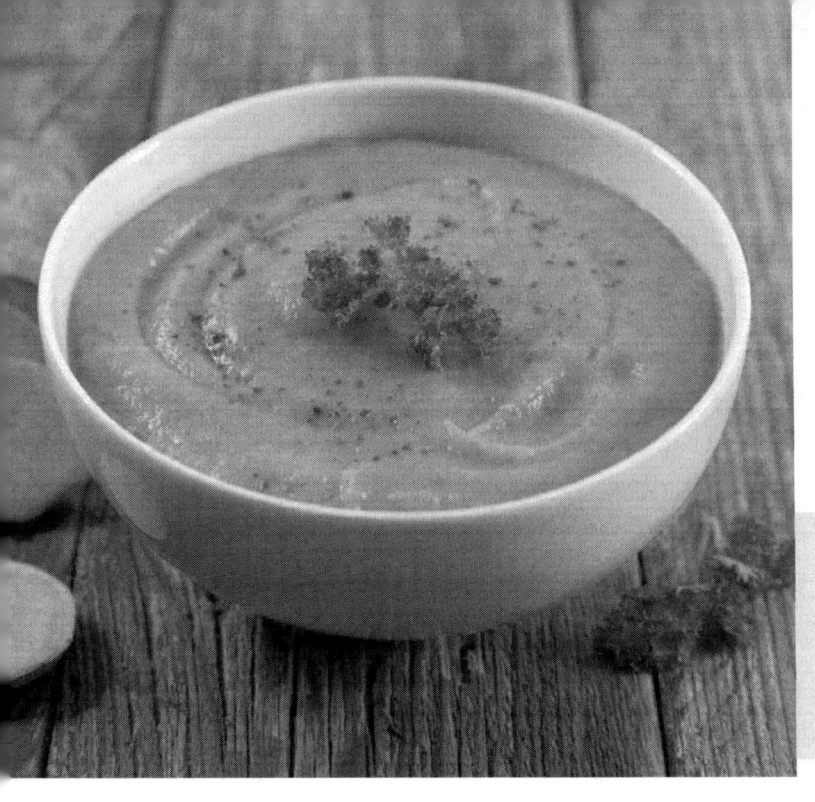

SWEET POTATO AND COCONUT SOUP

Anti-Inflammatory Benefits:
Sweet potatoes provide beta-carotene, while coconut milk contains healthy fats that reduce inflammation and support brain health.

PREP TIME: 10 MINS
COOK TIME: 20 MINS
SERVING: 3
Portion Size: 1 bowl per serving

INGREDIENTS

- 2 medium sweet potatoes (300 g), peeled and diced
- 1 cup (240 ml) coconut milk
- 1/2 onion (50 g), diced
- 2 cups (480 ml) vegetable broth
- 1/2 tsp (1 g) ground ginger
- 1 tbsp (15 ml) olive oil

EQUIPMENT NEEDED:
Pot, blender

INSTRUCTIONS

1. Heat one tbsp oil in a pot over moderate stove flame. Add chopped onion and softened for 3 minutes.
2. Toss in the sweet potatoes, vegetable broth, and ground ginger. Get it to a boil, then decrease the stove heat and simmer for 15 minutes until the sweet potatoes are tender.
3. Blend the soup on full power until the soup texture looks smooth using an immersion or regular blender.
4. Toss in the coconut milk, heat for 2 minutes, and serve warm.

NUTRITIONAL INFORMATION (PER SERVING):

Calories: 220 kcal, Carbohydrates: 28 g, Protein: 3 g, Fat: 10 g, Fiber: 5 g

HEALTH BENEFITS:

Seasonal Produce Swap: Use butternut squash or pumpkin instead of sweet potatoes.
Dietary Substitutions: Add a dash of cayenne pepper for a spicier flavor.

SUPERFOODS RECIPES

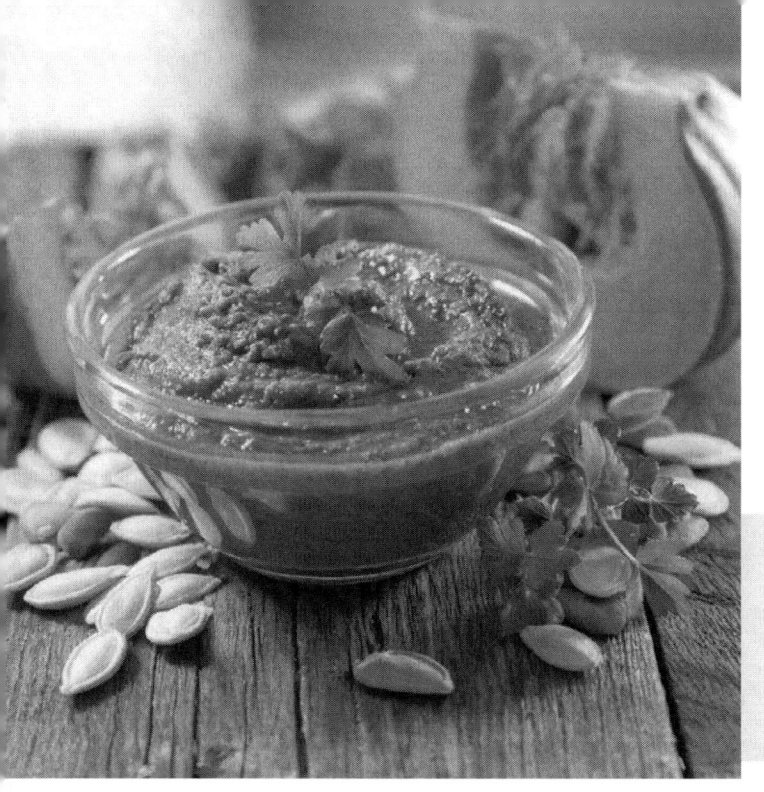

PUMPKIN SEED AND HERB PESTO

Anti-Inflammatory Benefits:
Pumpkin seeds are rich in magnesium and healthy fats, while fresh herbs provide antioxidants and anti-inflammatory properties.

PREP TIME: 5 MINS

COOK TIME: 00 MINS

SERVING: 4 Portion Size: 2 tbsp per serving

INGREDIENTS

- 1/4 cup (40 g) pumpkin seeds
- 1 cup (20 g) fresh basil leaves
- 1 clove garlic
- 1/4 cup (60 ml) olive oil
- 1 tbsp (15 ml) lemon juice
- Salt and pepper to taste

EQUIPMENT NEEDED:
Blender or food processor

INSTRUCTIONS

1. Combine all ingredients in a food blender. Blend on full power until the ingredient's texture looks smooth, scraping down the sides as needed.
2. Adjust the seasoning with salt and pepper.
3. Serve immediately as a sauce for pasta, vegetables, or as a spread.

NUTRITIONAL INFORMATION (PER SERVING):

Calories: 100 kcal, Carbohydrates: 2 g, Protein: 2 g, Fat: 10 g, Fiber: 1 g

HEALTH BENEFITS:
Seasonal Produce Swap: Use parsley or cilantro instead of basil.
Dietary Substitutions: Add nutritional yeast for a cheesy flavor without dairy.

BATCH COOKING

BATCH COOKING

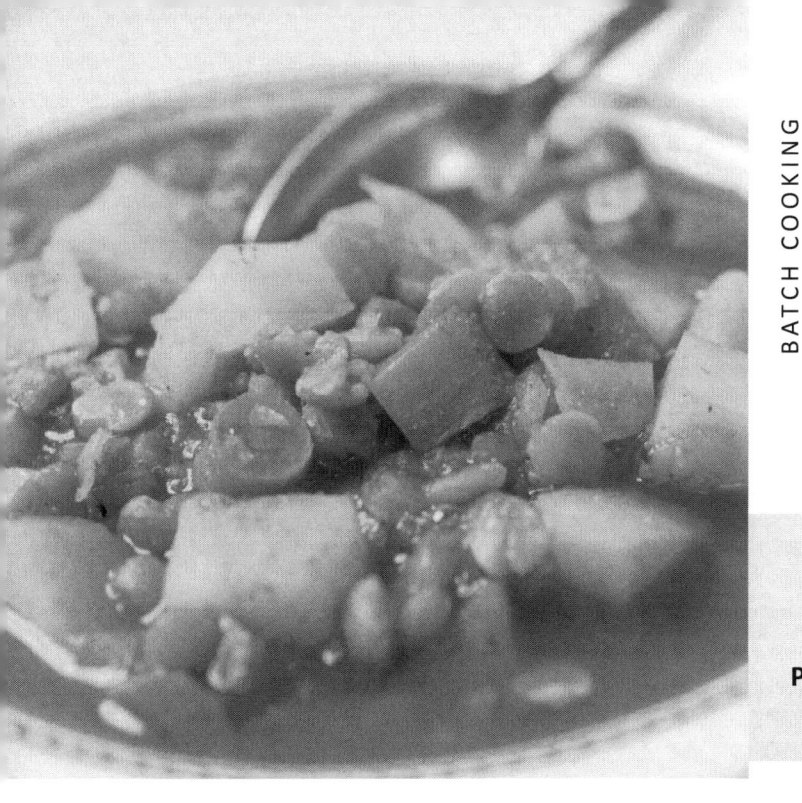

HEARTY VEGETABLE SOUP

Anti-Inflammatory Benefits:
Packed with a variety of vegetables, this soup is high in antioxidants, vitamins, and fiber to support immune health and reduce inflammation.

PREP TIME: 15 MINS
COOK TIME: 30 MINS
SERVING: 6 Portion Size: 1 bowl per serving

INGREDIENTS

- 1 cup (150 g) diced carrots
- 1 cup (100 g) diced celery
- 1 cup (100 g) diced zucchini
- 1 cup (150 g) diced tomatoes
- 2 cups (480 ml) vegetable broth
- 1/2 cup (75 g) green beans, chopped
- 1 tsp (2 g) dried thyme
- 1 tbsp (15 ml) olive oil
- Salt and pepper to taste

INSTRUCTIONS

1. Heat one tbsp oil in a pot over moderate stove flame. Add carrots and celery, and sauté for 5 minutes.
2. Toss in the zucchini, green beans, and tomatoes, cooking for another 3 minutes.
3. Add vegetable broth and dried thyme. Get it to a boil, then decrease the stove heat and simmer for 20 minutes.
4. Powder it with salt and crushed pepper, then serve warm.

EQUIPMENT NEEDED:
Large pot, spoon

NUTRITIONAL INFORMATION (PER SERVING):

Calories: 110 kcal, Carbohydrates: 15 g, Protein: 3 g, Fat: 4 g, Fiber: 5 g

HEALTH BENEFITS:
Seasonal Produce Swap: Add kale or spinach for extra greens.
Dietary Substitutions: Use chicken broth for added protein.

BLACK BEAN CHILI

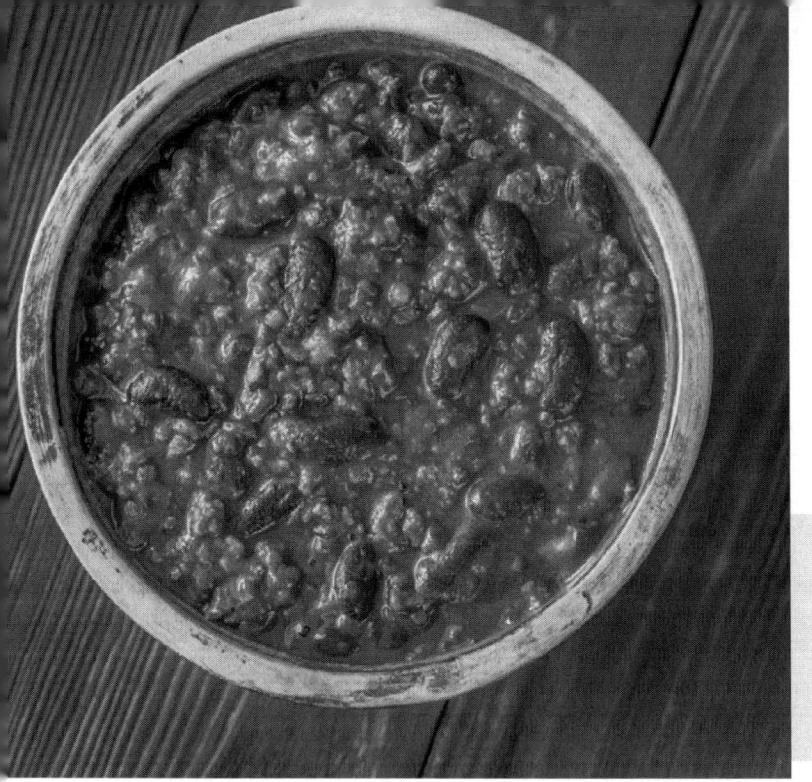

BATCH COOKING

Anti-Inflammatory Benefits:
Black beans provide plant-based protein and fiber, while spices like cumin and chili powder help reduce inflammation.

PREP TIME: 10 MINS

COOK TIME: 25 MINS

SERVING: 4
Portion Size: 1 bowl per serving

INGREDIENTS

- 1 cup (150 g) cooked black beans (or canned, drained and rinsed)
- 1 cup (150 g) diced tomatoes
- 1/2 cup (50 g) diced onion
- 1/2 cup (50 g) diced bell peppers
- 2 cups (480 ml) vegetable broth
- 1 tsp (2 g) ground cumin
- 1/2 tsp (1 g) chili powder
- 1 tbsp (15 ml) olive oil

EQUIPMENT NEEDED:
Large pot, spoon

INSTRUCTIONS

1. Heat one tbsp oil in a pot over moderate stove flame. Add chopped onion and bell peppers, and sauté for 5 minutes.
2. Toss in the black beans, diced tomatoes, vegetable broth, cumin, and chili powder.
3. Get it to a boil, then decrease the stove heat and simmer for 20 minutes.
4. Serve warm; spread fresh cilantro or avocado slices on top.

NUTRITIONAL INFORMATION (PER SERVING):

Calories: 180 kcal, Carbohydrates: 25 g, Protein: 8 g, Fat: 5 g, Fiber: 8 g

HEALTH BENEFITS:

Seasonal Produce Swap: Add zucchini or sweet corn in summer.
Dietary Substitutions: Replace black beans with kidney beans for variety.

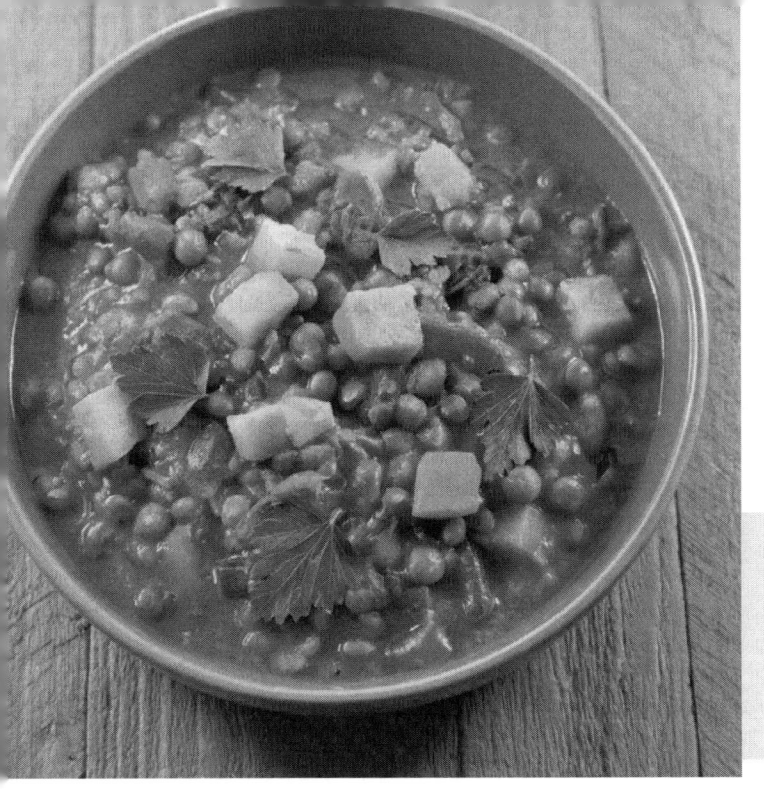

BATCH COOKING

LENTIL AND VEGETABLE CURRY

Anti-Inflammatory Benefits:
Lentils are rich in protein and fiber, while spices like turmeric and ginger provide powerful anti-inflammatory benefits.

PREP TIME: 10 MINS
COOK TIME: 25 MINS
SERVING: 4 Portion Size: 1 bowl per serving

INGREDIENTS

- 1 cup (150 g) cooked lentils
- 1 cup (150 g) diced tomatoes
- 1/2 cup (50 g) diced carrots
- 1/2 cup (50 g) diced zucchini
- 1 cup (240 ml) coconut milk
- 1 tsp (2 g) ground turmeric
- 1 tsp (2 g) grated ginger
- 1 tbsp (15 ml) olive oil

INSTRUCTIONS

1. Heat one tbsp oil in a pot over moderate stove flame. Add carrots and zucchini, and sauté for 5 minutes.
2. Toss in the lentils, tomatoes, coconut milk, turmeric, and ginger.
3. Get it to a simmer and cook for 15 minutes.
4. Serve warm with a side of whole-grain bread or rice.

EQUIPMENT NEEDED:
Pot, spoon

NUTRITIONAL INFORMATION (PER SERVING):

Calories: 220 kcal, Carbohydrates: 20 g, Protein: 7 g, Fat: 10 g, Fiber: 6 g

HEALTH BENEFITS:
Seasonal Produce Swap: Add butternut squash or sweet potato in autumn.
Dietary Substitutions: Replace coconut milk with almond milk for a lighter option.

BATCH COOKING

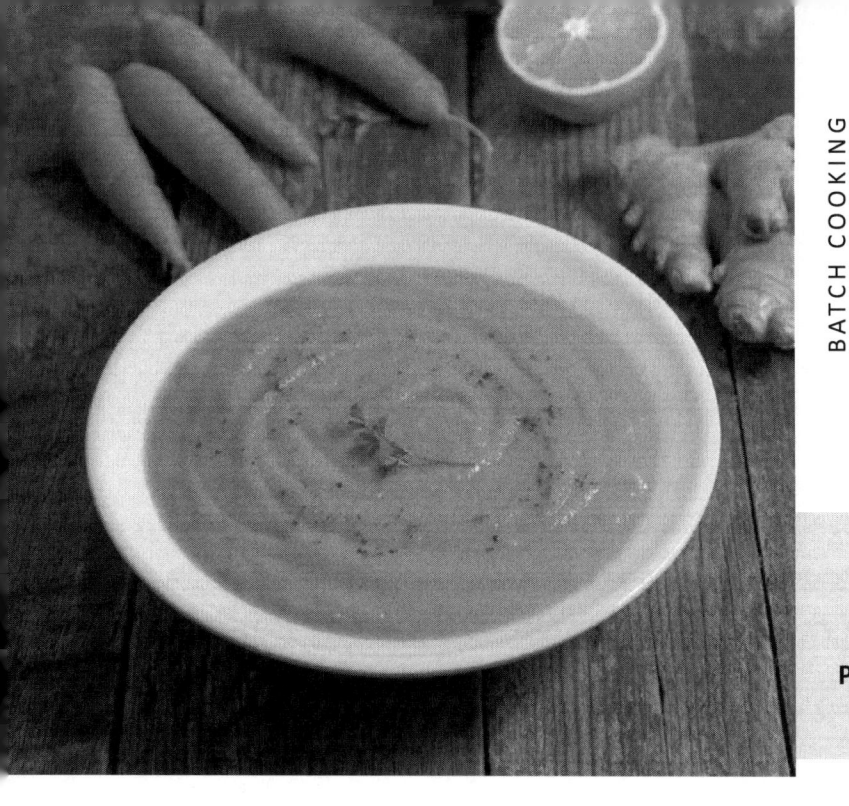

CARROT AND GINGER SOUP

Anti-Inflammatory Benefits:
Carrots are high in beta-carotene and antioxidants, while ginger helps reduce inflammation and supports digestion.

PREP TIME: 10 MINS
COOK TIME: 20 MINS
SERVING: 3
Portion Size: 1 bowl per serving

INGREDIENTS

- 2 cups (200 g) diced carrots
- 1/2 onion (50 g), diced
- 2 cups (480 ml) vegetable broth
- 1 tsp (2 g) grated ginger
- 1 tbsp (15 ml) olive oil
- Salt and pepper to taste

EQUIPMENT NEEDED:
Pot, blender

INSTRUCTIONS

1. Heat one tbsp oil in a pot over moderate stove flame. Add chopped onion and softened for 3 minutes.
2. Toss in the carrots, ginger, and vegetable broth. Get it to a boil, then decrease the stove heat and simmer for 15 minutes.
3. Blend the soup on full power until the soup texture looks smooth. Use an immersion or regular blender.
4. Powder it with salt and crushed pepper, then serve warm.

NUTRITIONAL INFORMATION (PER SERVING):

Calories: 100 kcal, Carbohydrates: 18 g, Protein: 2 g, Fat: 4 g, Fiber: 4 g

HEALTH BENEFITS:
Seasonal Produce Swap: Add parsnips or sweet potatoes for a sweeter flavor.
Dietary Substitutions: Use chicken broth for added protein.

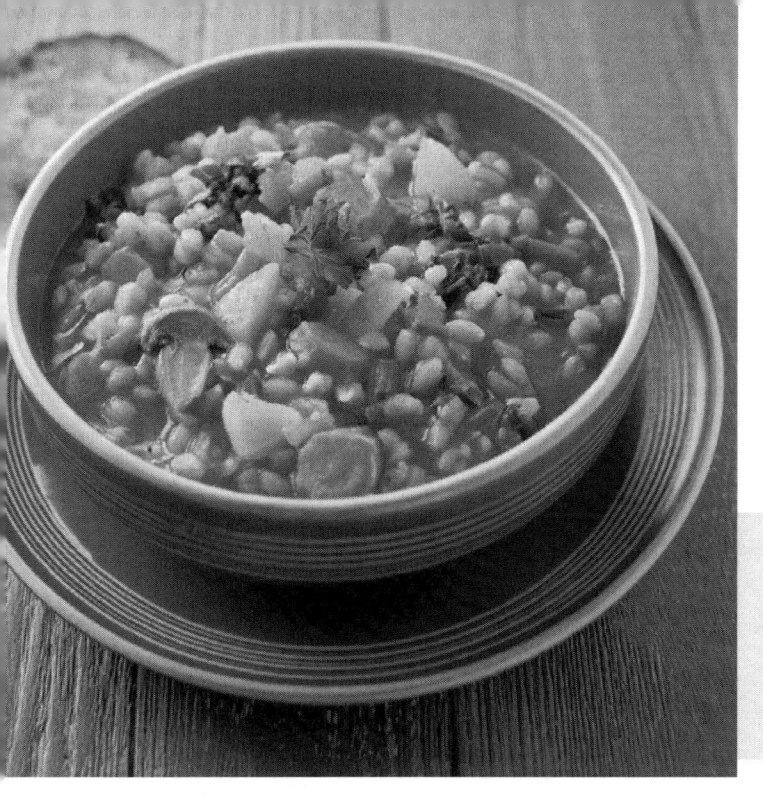

BATCH COOKING

VEGETABLE AND BARLEY STEW

Anti-Inflammatory Benefits:
Barley is rich in fiber, supporting gut health and reducing inflammation, while vegetables provide antioxidants and vitamins for immune support.

PREP TIME: 15 MINS

COOK TIME: 30 MINS

SERVING: 4
Portion Size: 1 bowl per serving

INGREDIENTS

- 1/2 cup (100 g) pearl barley
- 1 cup (100 g) diced carrots
- 1 cup (100 g) diced celery
- 1 cup (150 g) diced tomatoes
- 2 cups (480 ml) vegetable broth
- 1/2 tsp (1 g) dried thyme
- 1 tbsp (15 ml) olive oil
- Salt and pepper to taste

INSTRUCTIONS

1. Heat one tbsp oil in a pot over moderate stove flame. Add carrots and celery, and sauté for 5 minutes.
2. Toss in the barley, tomatoes, thyme, and vegetable broth.
3. Get it to a boil, then decrease the stove heat and simmer for 25–30 minutes until the barley is tender.
4. Powder it with salt and crushed pepper, then serve warm.

NUTRITIONAL INFORMATION (PER SERVING):

Calories: 180 kcal, Carbohydrates: 30 g, Protein: 5 g, Fat: 4 g, Fiber: 6 g

HEALTH BENEFITS:

Seasonal Produce Swap: Add green beans or zucchini for a summer twist. **Dietary Substitutions:** Use quinoa instead of barley for a gluten-free option.

EQUIPMENT NEEDED:

Large pot, spoon

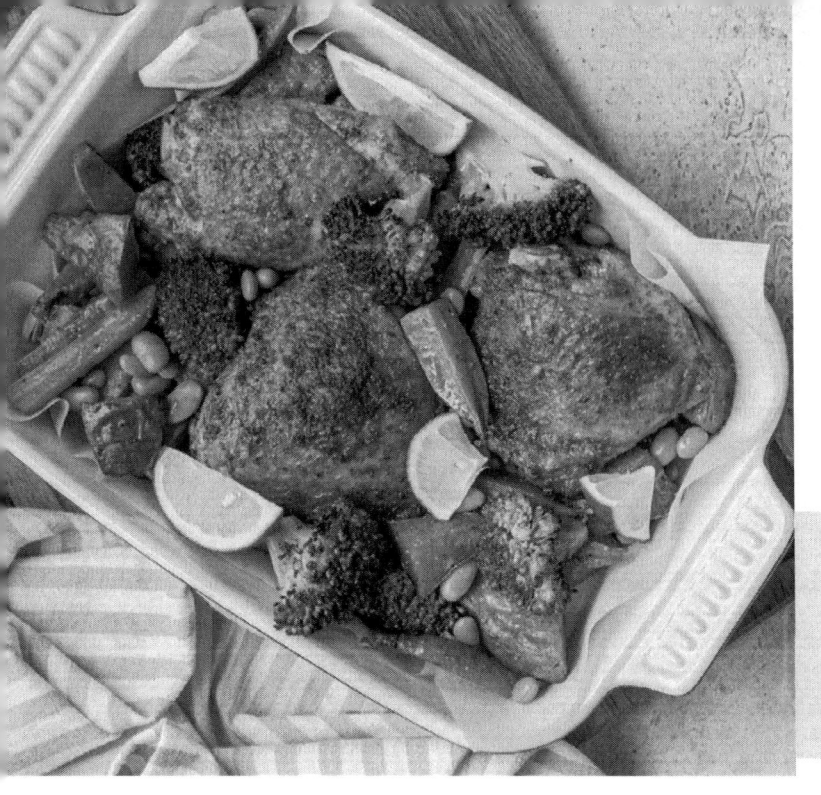

BATCH COOKING

BAKED CHICKEN THIGHS WITH ROOT VEGETABLES

Anti-Inflammatory Benefits:
Chicken thighs provide lean protein, while root vegetables like carrots and parsnips are rich in beta-carotene and other anti-inflammatory nutrients.

PREP TIME: 10 MINS

COOK TIME: 40 MINS

SERVING: 4
Portion Size: 1 chicken thigh and vegetables per serving

INGREDIENTS

- 4 bone-in chicken thighs (500 g total)
- 1 cup (150 g) diced carrots
- 1 cup (150 g) diced parsnips
- 1 tbsp (15 ml) olive oil
- 1 tsp (2 g) dried rosemary
- Salt and pepper to taste

INSTRUCTIONS

1. Preheat oven to 400°F (200°C).
2. Arrange the chicken thighs and vegetables on the paper-arranged baking sheet.
3. Drizzle one tbsp oil and sprinkle with rosemary, salt, and pepper.
4. Roast for 35–40 minutes, flip after the halftime has passed, until the chicken is fully cooked. Serve warm.

EQUIPMENT NEEDED:
Baking sheet, knife

NUTRITIONAL INFORMATION (PER SERVING):

Calories: 250 kcal, Carbohydrates: 10 g, Protein: 25 g, Fat: 12 g, Fiber: 3 g

HEALTH BENEFITS:
Seasonal Produce Swap: Replace parsnips with sweet potatoes or turnips.
Dietary Substitutions: Use tofu or tempeh as a plant-based alternative.

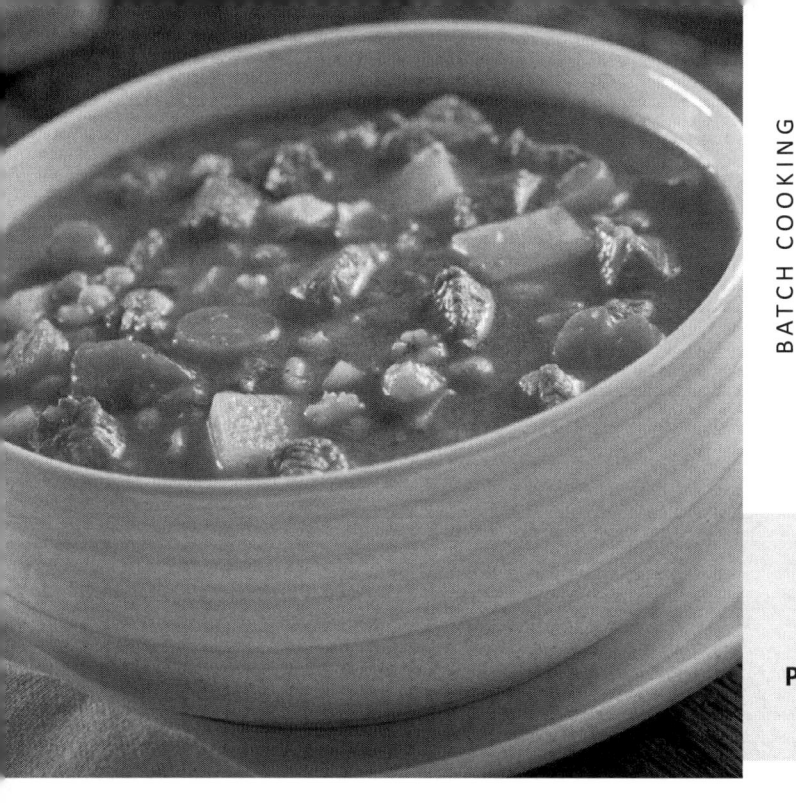

BEEF AND VEGETABLE STEW

BATCH COOKING

Anti-Inflammatory Benefits:
Beef is a high-quality protein source, while vegetables like carrots and celery provide antioxidants to reduce inflammation.

PREP TIME: 15 MINS
COOK TIME: 45 MINS
SERVING: 4 Portion Size: 1 bowl per serving

INGREDIENTS

- 500 g lean beef, diced
- 1 cup (100 g) diced carrots
- 1 cup (100 g) diced celery
- 1 cup (150 g) diced potatoes
- 2 cups (480 ml) beef broth
- 1/2 tsp (1 g) crushed black pepper
- 1 tbsp (15 ml) olive oil
- Salt to taste

EQUIPMENT NEEDED:
Large pot, spoon

INSTRUCTIONS

1. Heat one tbsp oil in a pot over moderate stove flame. Add meat pieces and cook until browned on all sides, about 5 minutes.
2. Toss in the carrots, celery, and potatoes, cooking for another 3 minutes.
3. Add beef broth and black pepper. Get it to a boil, then decrease the stove heat and simmer for 40 minutes or until the beef and vegetables are tender.
4. Season with salt, then serve warm.

NUTRITIONAL INFORMATION (PER SERVING):

Calories: 280 kcal, Carbohydrates: 18 g, Protein: 25 g, Fat: 10 g, Fiber: 4 g

HEALTH BENEFITS:
Seasonal Produce Swap: Add squash or turnips in autumn.
Dietary Substitutions: Replace beef with lentils for a vegetarian option.

MEDITERRANEAN EGGPLANT STEW

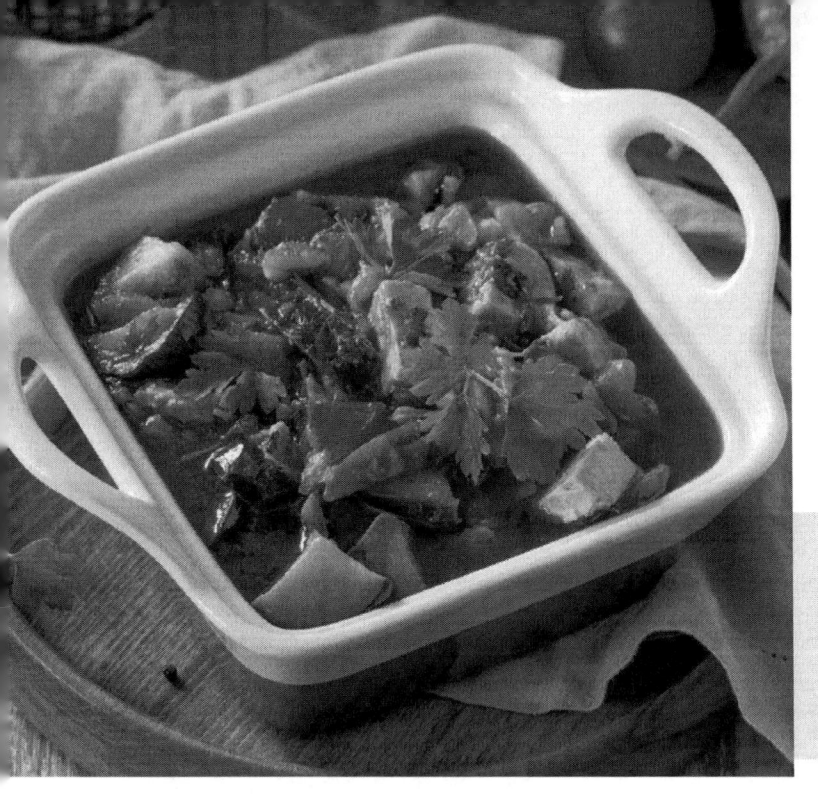

BATCH COOKING

Anti-Inflammatory Benefits:
Eggplant is rich in antioxidants like nasunin, while olive oil and tomatoes add heart-healthy fats and anti-inflammatory nutrients.

PREP TIME: 10 MINS

COOK TIME: 25 MINS

SERVING: 3
Portion Size: 1 bowl per serving

INGREDIENTS

- 1 medium eggplant (250 g), diced
- 1/2 cup (75 g) diced tomatoes
- 1/2 onion (50 g), diced
- 1/2 red bell pepper (50 g), diced
- 1 tbsp (15 ml) olive oil
- 1 tsp (2 g) dried oregano
- Salt and pepper to taste

INSTRUCTIONS

1. Heat one tbsp oil in a skillet over moderate stove flame. Add chopped onion and bell pepper, and sauté for 5 minutes.
2. Toss in the eggplant and cook for 10 minutes, until softened.
3. Add tomatoes and oregano, and simmer for another 10 minutes.
4. Powder it with salt and crushed pepper, then serve warm.

EQUIPMENT NEEDED:
Skillet, spoon

NUTRITIONAL INFORMATION (PER SERVING):

Calories: 140 kcal, Carbohydrates: 15 g, Protein: 3 g, Fat: 8 g, Fiber: 5 g

HEALTH BENEFITS:
Seasonal Produce Swap: Add zucchini or squash in summer.
Dietary Substitutions: Serve over quinoa or rice for a heartier meal.

FAMILY-FRIENDLY MEALS

FAMILY-FRIENDLY MEALS

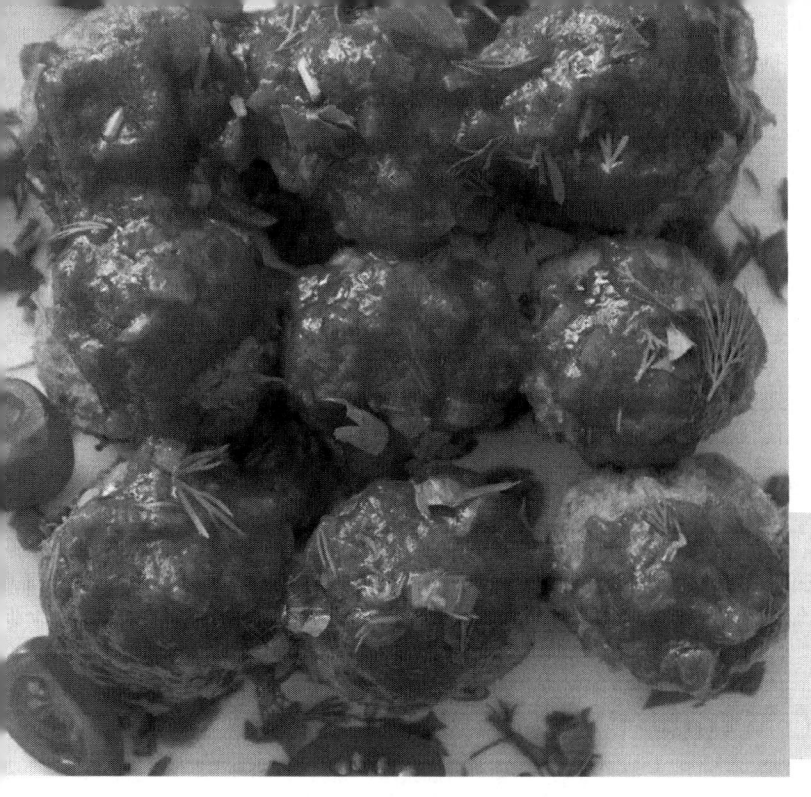

TURKEY AND VEGGIE MEATBALLS WITH TOMATO SAUCE

Anti-Inflammatory Benefits:
Turkey is a lean protein source, while the added vegetables and tomato sauce are rich in antioxidants that help reduce inflammation.

PREP TIME: 15 MINS

COOK TIME: 25 MINS

SERVING: 4
Portion Size: 3–4 meatballs per serving

INGREDIENTS

- 400 g ground turkey
- 1/2 cup (50 g) grated zucchini
- 1/2 cup (50 g) grated carrot
- 1/4 cup (30 g) breadcrumbs (or almond flour for a gluten-free option)
- 1 egg (50 g), beaten
- 1 tsp (2 g) dried oregano
- 1 tbsp (15 ml) olive oil
- 1 cup (240 ml) tomato sauce
- Salt and pepper to taste

EQUIPMENT NEEDED:
Mixing bowl, baking sheet, skillet

INSTRUCTIONS

1. Preheat oven to 375°F (190°C). Arrange the baking sheet with parchment paper.
2. Take a large, deep-bottom bowl and combine ground turkey, zucchini, carrot, breadcrumbs, egg, oregano, salt, and pepper. Mix until well combined.
3. Form the mixture into small meatballs and place them on the paper-arranged baking sheet.
4. Bake for 17–20 minutes so the meatballs get the golden brown color and fully cooked.
5. Meanwhile, heat one tbsp oil in a skillet over moderate stove flame. Add tomato sauce and get it simmer over low flame for 5 minutes.
6. Add baked meatballs to the sauce, toss to coat, and serve warm.

NUTRITIONAL INFORMATION (PER SERVING):

Calories: 220 kcal, Carbohydrates: 10 g, Protein: 25 g, Fat: 8 g, Fiber: 2 g

HEALTH BENEFITS:
Seasonal Produce Swap: Add chopped spinach or kale for extra nutrients.
Dietary Substitutions: Replace turkey with chicken or beef or use chickpeas for a vegetarian option.

FAMILY-FRIENDLY MEALS

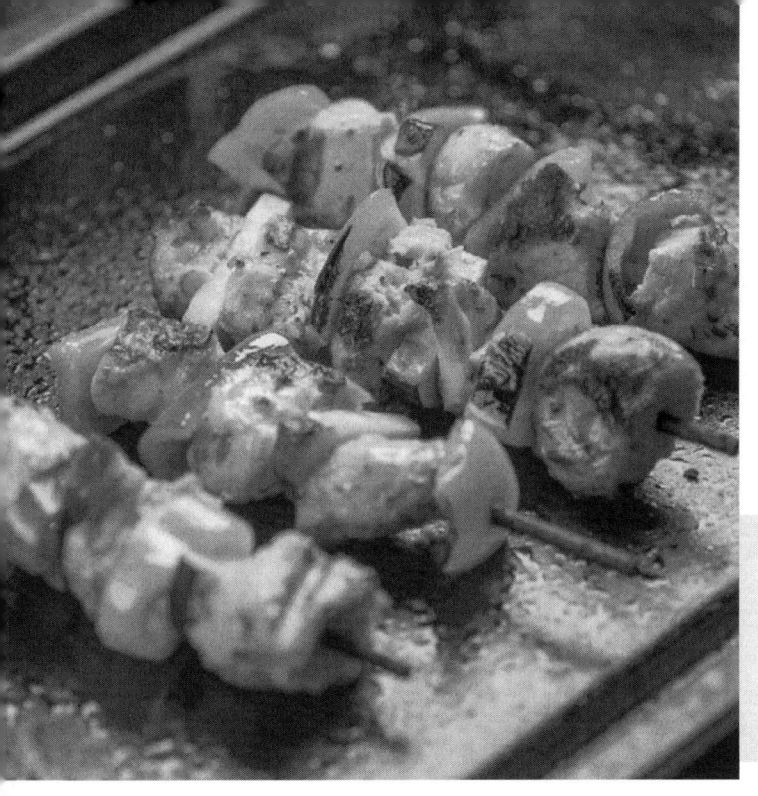

CHICKEN AND VEGGIE SKEWERS

Anti-Inflammatory Benefits:
Chicken provides lean protein, and vegetables like bell peppers and zucchini are high in antioxidants and vitamins.

PREP TIME: 15 MINS

COOK TIME: 10 MINS

SERVING: 4
Portion Size: 2 skewers per serving

INGREDIENTS

- 400 g boneless, skinless chicken breast, cubed
- 1 cup (100 g) zucchini, sliced
- 1 cup (100 g) red bell pepper, diced
- 1/2 cup (50 g) red onion, diced
- 1 tbsp (15 ml) olive oil
- 1 tsp (2 g) dried Italian herbs
- Salt and pepper to taste

INSTRUCTIONS

1. Preheat grill or grill pan.
2. Take a deep-bottom bowl and toss chicken cubes and vegetables with olive oil, Italian herbs, salt, and pepper.
3. Thread the chicken and veggies on skewers, alternating ingredients.
4. Grill for 8–10 minutes, turning in 2 minutes time intervals, until the meat is done properly and the vegetables are slightly charred.
5. Serve warm with a side of quinoa or a green salad.

EQUIPMENT NEEDED:
Skewers, grill, or grill pan

NUTRITIONAL INFORMATION (PER SERVING):

Calories: 180 kcal, Carbohydrates: 5 g, Protein: 28 g, Fat: 5 g, Fiber: 2 g

HEALTH BENEFITS:
Seasonal Produce Swap: Use asparagus or cherry tomatoes in spring.
Dietary Substitutions: Replace chicken with tofu or shrimp for variety.

FAMILY-FRIENDLY MEALS

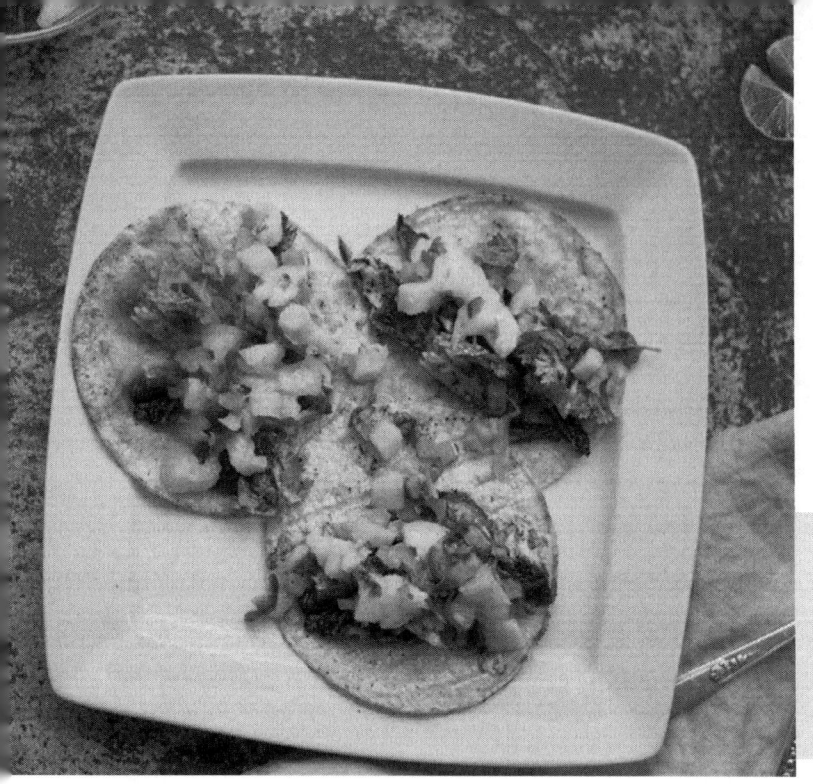

FISH TACOS WITH MANGO SALSA

Anti-Inflammatory Benefits:
Fishlike cod or tilapia is a lean protein, while mango provides vitamin C and antioxidants to reduce inflammation.

PREP TIME: 15 MINS

COOK TIME: 10 MINS

SERVING: 4
Portion Size: 2 tacos per serving

INGREDIENTS

- 200 g white fish fillets (cod or tilapia)
- 4 small corn tortillas
- 1 cup (150 g) diced mango
- 1/4 cup (40 g) diced red onion
- 1/4 cup (10 g) fresh cilantro, chopped
- 1 tbsp (15 ml) lime juice
- 1 tsp (2 g) ground cumin
- 1 tbsp (15 ml) olive oil
- Salt and pepper to taste

EQUIPMENT NEEDED:
Skillet, knife

INSTRUCTIONS

1. Take a deep-bottom bowl and combine mango, red onion, cilantro, lime juice, salt, and crushed pepper to make the mango salsa. Set aside.
2. Season the fish with cumin, salt, and pepper.
3. Heat one tbsp oil in a skillet over moderate stove flame. Cook the fish for 3–4 minutes on one side until flaky and fully cooked.
4. Warm the tortillas.
5. Assemble the tacos with fish over tortillas and topping them with mango salsa. Serve immediately.

NUTRITIONAL INFORMATION (PER SERVING):

Calories: 220 kcal, Carbohydrates: 20 g, Protein: 20 g, Fat: 7 g, Fiber: 4 g

HEALTH BENEFITS:

Seasonal Produce Swap: Substitute mango with pineapple or peach in summer.
Dietary Substitutions: Use lettuce wraps instead of tortillas for a low-carb option.

FAMILY-FRIENDLY MEALS

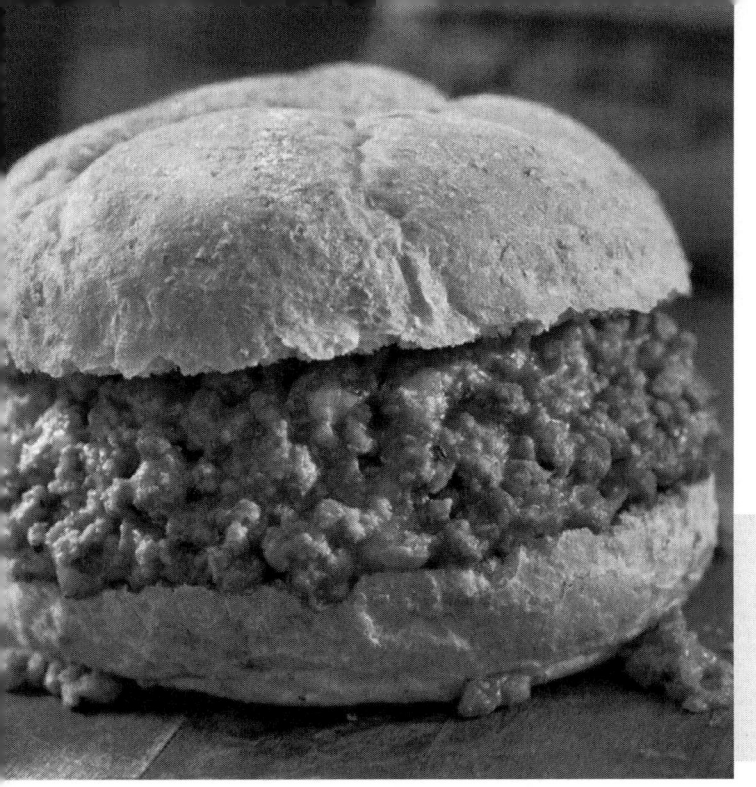

SLOPPY JOES WITH LENTILS

Anti-Inflammatory Benefits:
Lentils are high in fiber and plant-based protein, while spices like paprika and cumin provide anti-inflammatory properties.

PREP TIME: 10 MINS

COOK TIME: 20 MINS

SERVING: 4
Portion Size: 1 sandwich per serving

INGREDIENTS

- 1 cup (150 g) cooked lentils
- 1/2 cup (75 g) diced tomatoes
- 1/4 cup (40 g) diced onion
- 1/4 cup (40 g) diced bell pepper
- 1 tbsp (15 ml) tomato paste
- 1 tsp (2 g) smoked paprika
- 1/2 tsp (1 g) ground cumin
- 4 whole-grain buns
- 1 tbsp (15 ml) olive oil

INSTRUCTIONS

1. Heat one tbsp oil in a skillet over moderate stove flame. Add chopped onion and diced bell pepper, and sauté for 3 minutes.
2. Toss in the lentils, tomatoes, tomato paste, paprika, cumin, salt, and pepper. Cook for 10 minutes, keep stirring occasionally, until the mixture thickens.
3. Toast the whole-grain buns and spoon the lentil mixture onto the bottom halves.
4. Place the top halves of the buns and serve warm.

NUTRITIONAL INFORMATION (PER SERVING):

Calories: 200 kcal, Carbohydrates: 30 g, Protein: 8 g, Fat: 4 g, Fiber: 8 g

HEALTH BENEFITS:
Seasonal Produce Swap: Add zucchini or corn in summer.
Dietary Substitutions: Use gluten-free buns or serve over rice for a different option.

EQUIPMENT NEEDED:
Skillet, spoon

FAMILY-FRIENDLY MEALS

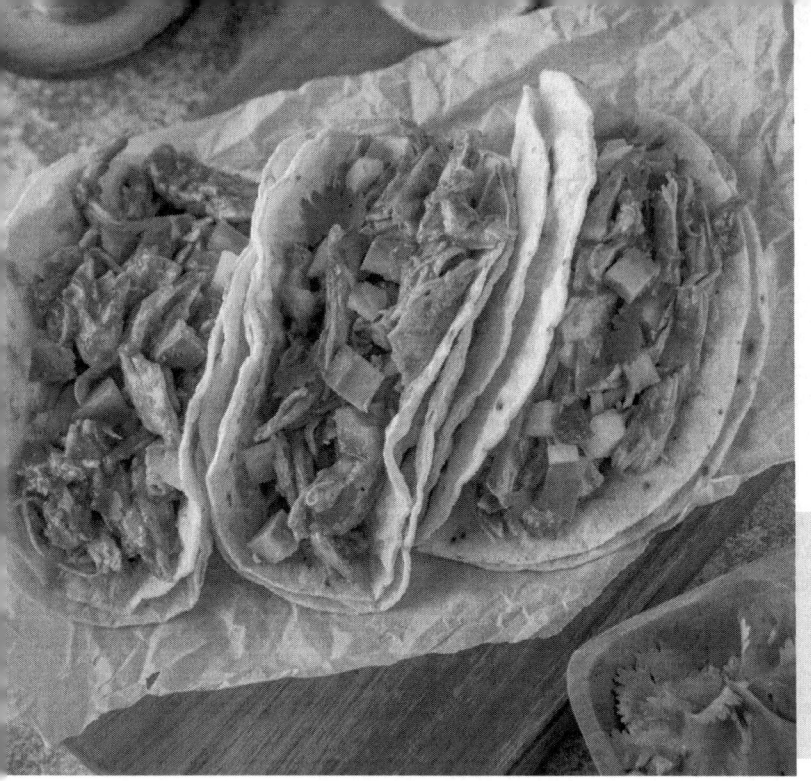

MINI CHICKEN AND AVOCADO TACOS

Anti-Inflammatory Benefits:
Chicken is a lean protein source, while avocados provide anti-inflammatory monounsaturated fats and essential nutrients.

PREP TIME: 15 MINS

COOK TIME: 10 MINS

SERVING: 4
Portion Size: 2 tacos per serving

INGREDIENTS

- 200 g boneless, skinless chicken breast, diced
- 1/2 tsp (1 g) ground cumin
- 1/2 tsp (1 g) paprika
- 1 tbsp (15 ml) olive oil
- 8 mini corn tortillas
- 1 avocado (150 g), diced
- 1/4 cup (40 g) diced red onion
- 1 tbsp (15 ml) lime juice
- Salt and pepper to taste

EQUIPMENT NEEDED:
Skillet, knife, mixing bowl

INSTRUCTIONS

1. Heat one tbsp oil in a skillet over moderate stove flame. Season the chicken with cumin, paprika, salt, and pepper. Cook for 7–10 minutes, stirring occasionally, until fully cooked.
2. Take a large deep-bottom bowl and combine the avocado, diced red onion, lime juice, salt, and crushed pepper to make a simple avocado salsa.
3. Warm the tortillas.
4. Fill each tortilla with cooked chicken and top with avocado salsa. Serve immediately.

NUTRITIONAL INFORMATION (PER SERVING):

Calories: 250 kcal, Carbohydrates: 20 g, Protein: 20 g, Fat: 10 g, Fiber: 5 g

HEALTH BENEFITS:
Seasonal Produce Swap: Add fresh corn or diced tomatoes in summer.
Dietary Substitutions: Use lettuce wraps instead of tortillas for a low-carb option.

FAMILY-FRIENDLY MEALS

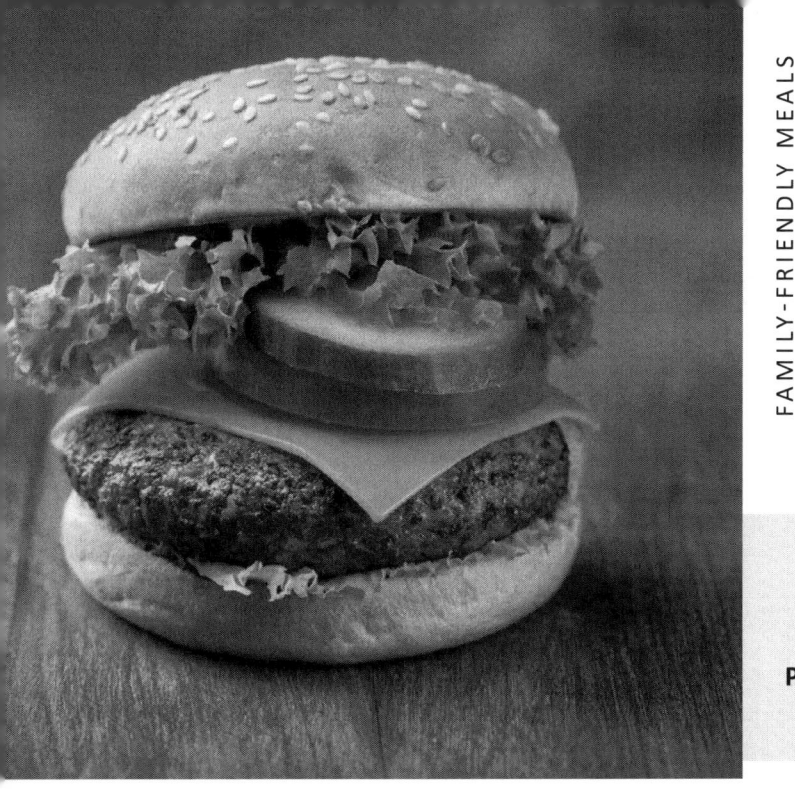

BEEF AND VEGGIE BURGERS

Anti-Inflammatory Benefits:
Lean beef provides high-quality protein, while vegetables like zucchini and carrots add fiber and antioxidants to reduce inflammation.

PREP TIME: 15 MINS

COOK TIME: 10 MINS

SERVING: 4
Portion Size: 1 burger per serving

INGREDIENTS

- 400 g lean ground beef
- 1/4 cup (30 g) grated zucchini
- 1/4 cup (30 g) grated carrot
- 1/4 cup (30 g) breadcrumbs (or almond flour for gluten-free)
- 1 tsp (2 g) garlic powder
- 1 tbsp (15 ml) olive oil
- 4 whole-grain burger buns
- Salt and pepper to taste

EQUIPMENT NEEDED:
Skillet or grill pan, mixing bowl

INSTRUCTIONS

1. Take a large, deep-bottom bowl and combine ground beef, zucchini, carrot, breadcrumbs, garlic powder, salt, and pepper. Mix until well combined.
2. Form the mixture into 4 patties.
3. Heat one tbsp oil in a skillet or grill pan over moderate stove flame. Cook the patties for 4–5 minutes on one side or until fully cooked.
4. Toast the burger buns and assemble them with patties and your choice of toppings like lettuce, tomato, or avocado. Serve warm.

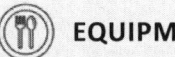

NUTRITIONAL INFORMATION (PER SERVING):

Calories: 280 kcal, Carbohydrates: 22 g, Protein: 22 g, Fat: 10 g, Fiber: 4 g

HEALTH BENEFITS:
Seasonal Produce Swap: Add grilled zucchini or mushrooms in summer.
Dietary Substitutions: Use lettuce wraps instead of buns for a low-carb option.

FAMILY-FRIENDLY MEALS

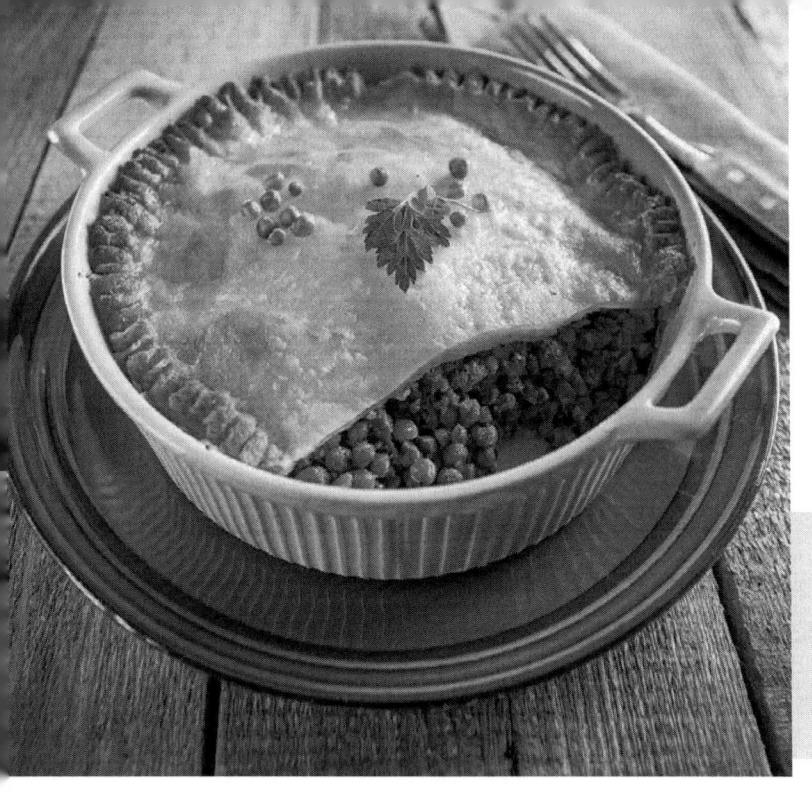

SHEPHERD'S PIE WITH LENTILS

Anti-Inflammatory Benefits:
Lentils are a great source of plant-based protein and fiber, while sweet potatoes provide beta-carotene and antioxidants.

PREP TIME: 15 MINS

COOK TIME: 30 MINS

SERVING: 4
1 portion per serving

INGREDIENTS

- 1 cup (150 g) cooked lentils
- 1 cup (100 g) diced carrots
- 1/2 cup (50 g) diced onion
- 1/2 cup (50 g) green peas
- 1 cup (200 g) mashed sweet potatoes
- 1 tbsp (15 ml) olive oil
- 1 tsp (2 g) dried thyme
- Salt and pepper to taste

EQUIPMENT NEEDED:
Baking dish, pot, skillet

INSTRUCTIONS

1. Preheat oven to 375°F (190°C).
2. Heat one tbsp oil in a skillet over moderate stove flame. Add carrots and onion, and sauté for 5 minutes. Toss in lentils, peas, thyme, salt, and pepper. Cook for 5 minutes.
3. Transfer the lentil mixture to the paper-arranged baking dish and spread the sweet potatoes on top.
4. Bake for 17-20 minutes, until golden and bubbly. Serve warm.

NUTRITIONAL INFORMATION (PER SERVING):

Calories: 220 kcal, Carbohydrates: 32 g, Protein: 7 g, Fat: 6 g, Fiber: 8 g

HEALTH BENEFITS:

Seasonal Produce Swap: Add parsnips or butternut squash in autumn.
Dietary Substitutions: Use mashed cauliflower instead of sweet potatoes for a lower-carb option.

FAMILY-FRIENDLY MEALS

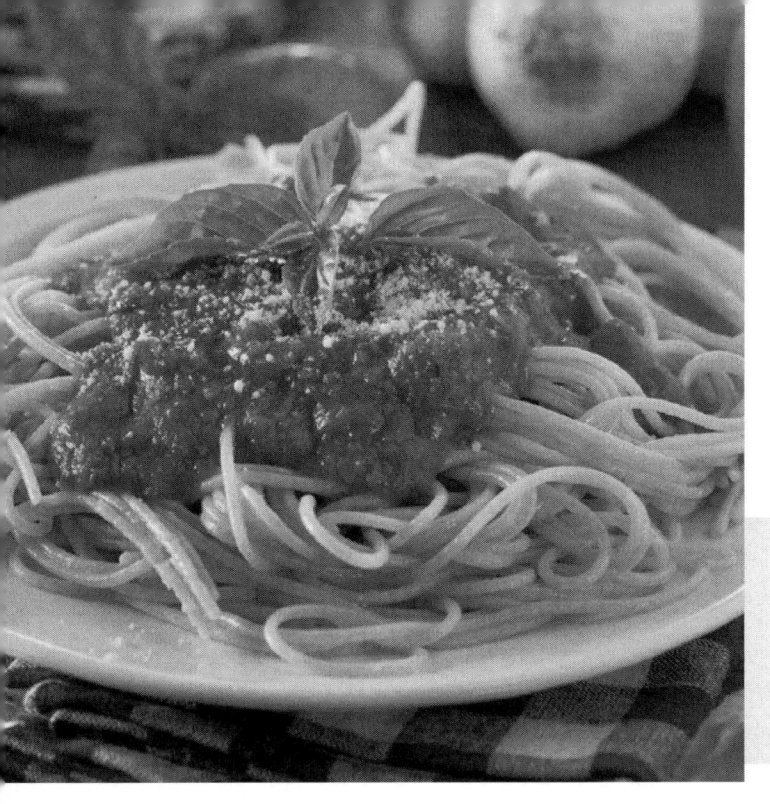

SPAGHETTI SQUASH MARINARA

Anti-Inflammatory Benefits:
Spaghetti squash is a low-carb alternative to pasta, and the marinara sauce is rich in lycopene and other anti-oxidants.

PREP TIME: 10 MINS

COOK TIME: 40 MINS

SERVING: 4
Portion Size: 1 bowl per serving

INGREDIENTS

- 1 medium spaghetti squash (800 g)
- 2 cups (480 ml) marinara sauce
- 1/4 cup (10 g) basil leaves, chopped
- 1 tbsp (15 ml) olive oil
- Salt and pepper to taste

INSTRUCTIONS

1. Preheat oven to 375°F (190°C). Slice the spaghetti squash in half lengthwise to discard the seeds. Drizzle one tbsp oil and powder it with salt and crushed pepper.
2. Place the squash halves on the parchment paper-arranged baking sheet and roast for 37–40 minutes.
3. Meanwhile, heat the marinara sauce in a skillet over moderate stove flame.
4. Once cooked, use a fork to scrape squash spaghetti flesh into strands.
5. Divide the squash among bowls, top with marinara sauce, and spread fresh basil on top. Serve warm.

NUTRITIONAL INFORMATION (PER SERVING):

Calories: 160 kcal, Carbohydrates: 20 g, Protein: 3 g, Fat: 7 g, Fiber: 4 g

HEALTH BENEFITS:
Seasonal Produce Swap: Add sautéed mushrooms or spinach to the marinara sauce.
Dietary Substitutions: Use zucchini noodles instead of spaghetti squash.

EQUIPMENT NEEDED:
Baking sheet, fork, skillet

JAPANESE & MEDITERRANEAN

JAPANESE & MEDITERRANEAN RECIPES

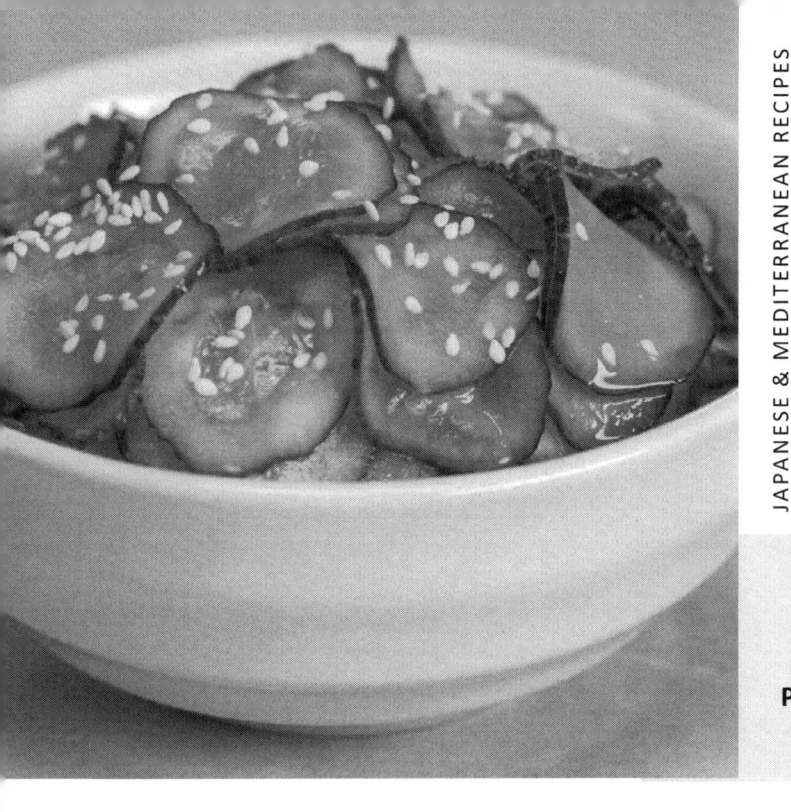

JAPANESE CUCUMBER SALAD

Anti-Inflammatory Benefits:
Cucumbers are hydrating and contain antioxidants, while rice vinegar provides anti-inflammatory properties.

PREP TIME: 10 MINS
COOK TIME: 00 MINS
SERVING: 2
Portion Size: 1 bowl per serving

INGREDIENTS

- 1 large cucumber (200 g), thinly sliced
- 1 tbsp (15 ml) rice vinegar
- 1 tsp (5 ml) sesame oil
- 1 tsp (5 g) sesame seeds
- 1/2 tsp (2 g) sugar or honey (optional)
- Pinch of salt

EQUIPMENT NEEDED:
Knife, mixing bowl

INSTRUCTIONS

1. Take a large deep-bottom bowl and combine rice vinegar, sesame oil, sugar (if using), and a pinch of salt. Stir until sugar dissolves.
2. Add cucumber slices and toss to coat evenly. Sprinkle with sesame seeds and serve immediately.

NUTRITIONAL INFORMATION (PER SERVING):

Calories: 60 kcal, Carbohydrates: 4 g, Protein: 1 g, Fat: 4 g, Fiber: 1 g

HEALTH BENEFITS:
Seasonal Produce Swap: Add sliced radishes for extra crunch.
Dietary Substitutions: Use maple syrup instead of sugar for a vegan option.

JAPANESE & MEDITERRANEAN RECIPES

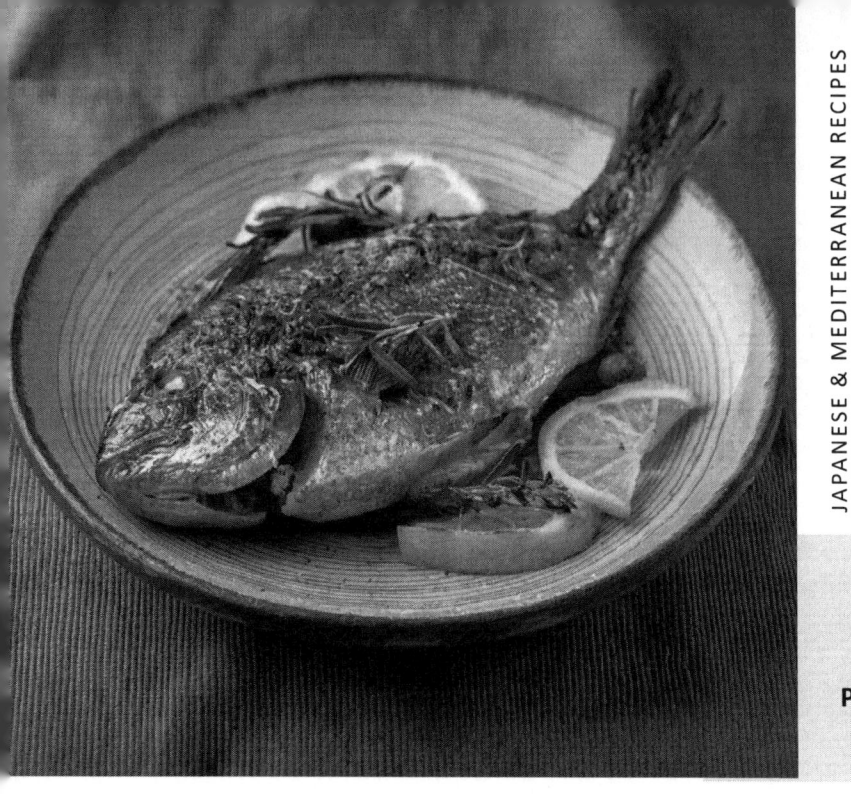

MEDITERRANEAN BAKED FISH WITH HERBS

Anti-Inflammatory Benefits:
Fish is rich in omega-3 fatty acids, while Mediterranean herbs provide antioxidants and anti-inflammatory compounds.

PREP TIME: 10 MINS

COOK TIME: 20 MINS

SERVING: 2
Portion Size: 1 fillet per serving

INGREDIENTS

- 2 white fish fillets (300 g total, such as cod or sea bass)
- 1 tbsp (15 ml) olive oil
- 1 tsp (2 g) dried oregano
- 1 tsp (2 g) dried thyme
- 1/4 cup (10 g) fresh parsley, chopped
- 2 lemon slices
- Salt and pepper to taste

EQUIPMENT NEEDED:
Baking dish, aluminum foil

INSTRUCTIONS

1. Preheat oven to 375°F (190°C).
2. Place the fillets on the foil sheet-arranged baking dish. Drizzle one tbsp oil and sprinkle with oregano, thyme, salt, and pepper.
3. Top each fillet with a lemon slice and sprinkle with fresh parsley.
4. Fold the foil to make the sealed packet and bake for 20 minutes until the fillet flakes easily.
5. Serve immediately.

NUTRITIONAL INFORMATION (PER SERVING):

Calories: 180 kcal, Carbohydrates: 1 g, Protein: 30 g, Fat: 7 g, Fiber: 0 g

HEALTH BENEFITS:
Seasonal Produce Swap: Add cherry tomatoes or zucchini slices to the baking dish.
Dietary Substitutions: Use salmon instead of white fish for a richer flavor.

JAPANESE & MEDITERRANEAN RECIPES

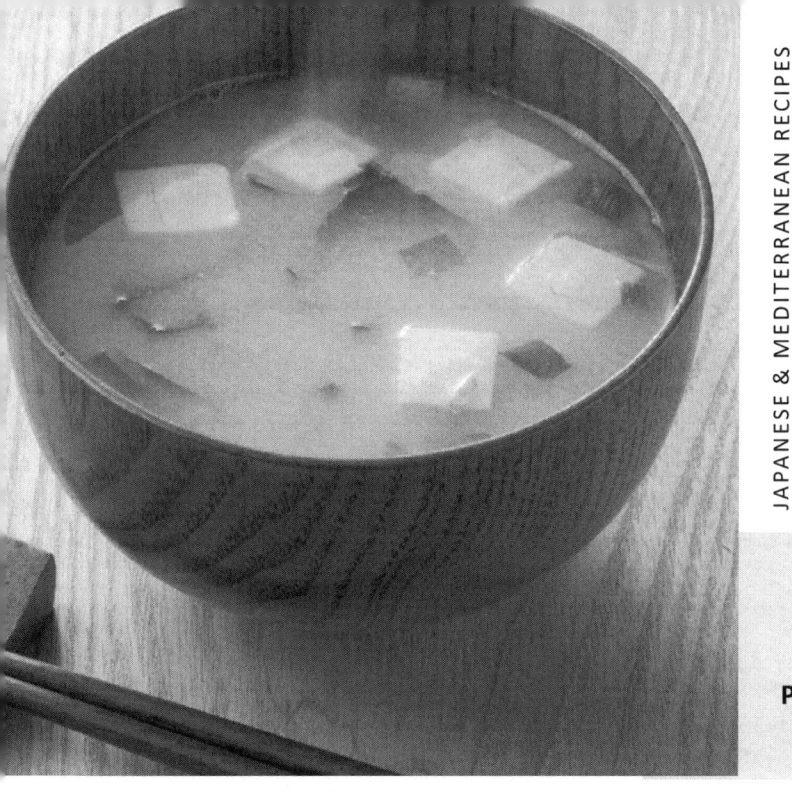

MISO SOUP WITH SEAWEED AND TOFU

Anti-Inflammatory Benefits:
Miso is a fermented food rich in probiotics, while seaweed provides iodine and antioxidants to reduce inflammation.

PREP TIME: 5 MINS
COOK TIME: 10 MINS
SERVING: 3
Portion Size: 1 bowl per serving

INGREDIENTS

- 3 cups (720 ml) water
- 2 tbsp (30 g) miso paste
- 1/2 cup (100 g) tofu, cubed
- 1/4 cup (10 g) dried seaweed (wakame)
- 1/4 cup (10 g) green onions, sliced

INSTRUCTIONS

1. Heat water in a pot over a moderate stove flame until it begins to simmer.
2. Toss in the miso paste until fully dissolved.
3. Add tofu and seaweed, and simmer for 5 minutes. Spread sliced green onions on top before serving.

EQUIPMENT NEEDED:
Pot, ladle

NUTRITIONAL INFORMATION (PER SERVING):

Calories: 80 kcal, Carbohydrates: 6 g, Protein: 6 g, Fat: 3 g, Fiber: 1 g

HEALTH BENEFITS:
Seasonal Produce Swap: Add mushrooms or spinach for extra nutrients.
Dietary Substitutions: Use chickpea miso for a soy-free option.

JAPANESE & MEDITERRANEAN RECIPES

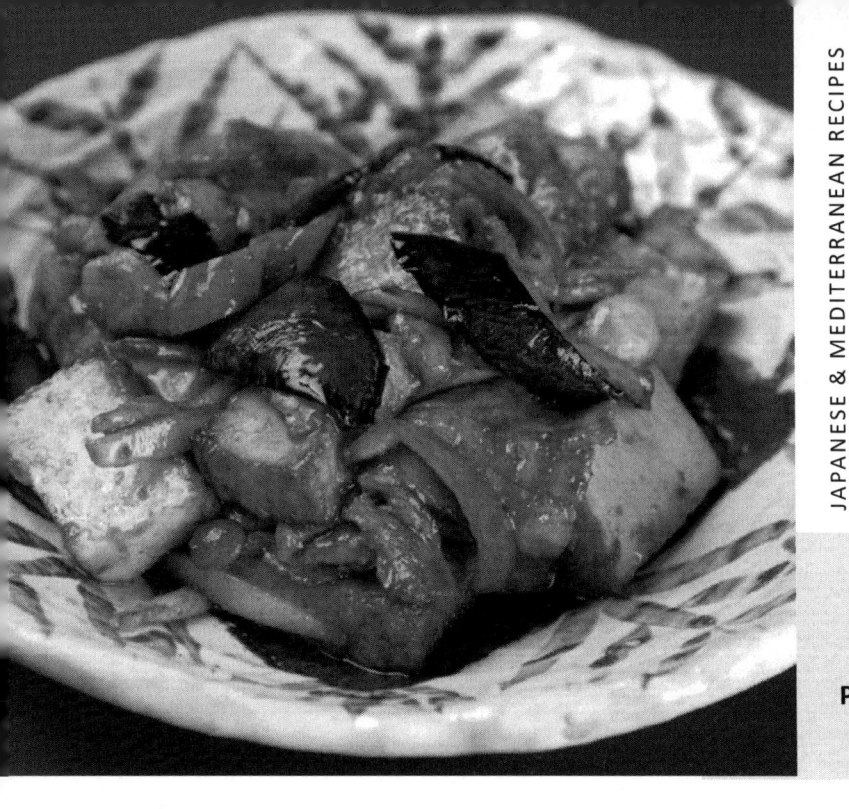

JAPANESE EGGPLANT STIR-FRY

Anti-Inflammatory Benefits:
Eggplants are high in antioxidants like nasunin, while sesame oil adds anti-inflammatory fats.

PREP TIME: 10 MINS

COOK TIME: 10 MINS

SERVING: 3
Portion Size: 1 bowl per serving

INGREDIENTS

- 2 small Japanese eggplants (250 g), sliced
- 1 tbsp (15 ml) sesame oil
- 1 tbsp (15 ml) soy sauce (low sodium)
- 1 tsp (5 ml) rice vinegar
- 1 clove garlic, minced
- 1 tsp (2 g) sesame seeds

INSTRUCTIONS

1. Heat one tbsp sesame oil in a skillet over moderate stove flame. Add garlic and sauté for 1 minute until fragrant.
2. Add sliced eggplants and cook for 7–8 minutes, stirring occasionally, until tender.
3. Toss in the soy sauce and rice vinegar and cook for 1 minute.
4. Sprinkle with sesame seeds and serve warm.

EQUIPMENT NEEDED:
Skillet, spatula

NUTRITIONAL INFORMATION (PER SERVING):

Calories: 120 kcal, Carbohydrates: 10 g, Protein: 2 g, Fat: 8 g, Fiber: 4 g

HEALTH BENEFITS:
Seasonal Produce Swap: Add zucchini or bell peppers for variety.
Dietary Substitutions: Use tamari instead of soy sauce for a gluten-free option.

MEDITERRANEAN CHICKPEA STEW

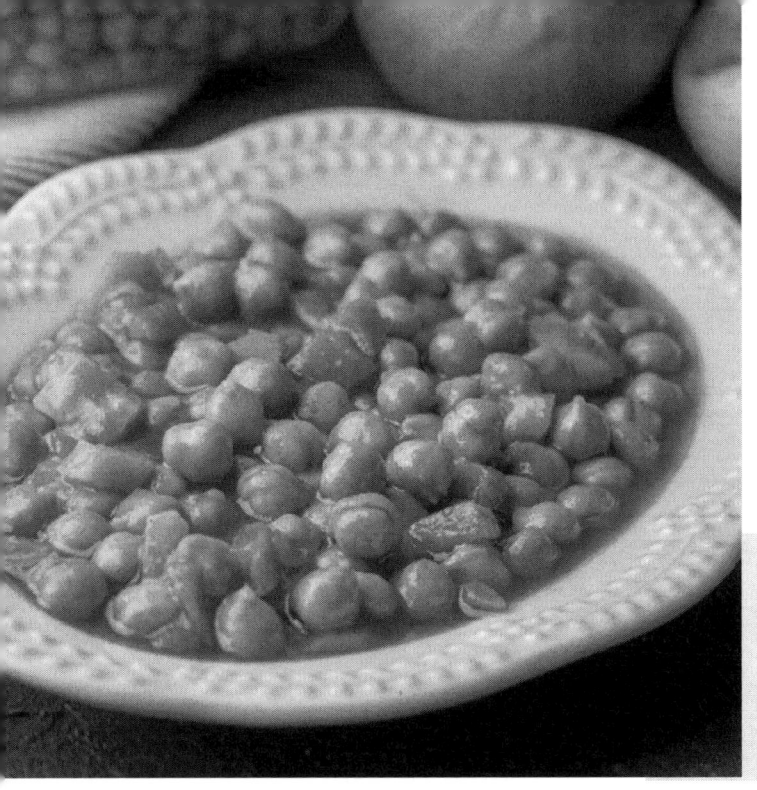

JAPANESE & MEDITERRANEAN RECIPES

Anti-Inflammatory Benefits:
Chickpeas are a great source of plant-based protein and fiber, while tomatoes and olive oil add heart-healthy antioxidants.

PREP TIME: 10 MINS

COOK TIME: 20 MINS

SERVING: 3
Portion Size: 1 bowl per serving

INGREDIENTS

- 1 cup (150 g) cooked chickpeas
- 1 cup (150 g) diced tomatoes
- 1/2 cup (50 g) diced onion
- 1/4 cup (10 g) fresh parsley, chopped
- 1 tbsp (15 ml) olive oil
- 1/2 tsp (1 g) ground cumin
- Salt and pepper to taste

EQUIPMENT NEEDED:
Pot, spoon

INSTRUCTIONS

1. Heat one tbsp oil in a pot over moderate stove flame. Add chopped onion and softened for 3 minutes.
2. Toss in the chickpeas, tomatoes, cumin, salt, and pepper. Simmer for 15 minutes.
3. Spread fresh parsley on top and serve warm with a side of whole-grain bread.

NUTRITIONAL INFORMATION (PER SERVING):

Calories: 180 kcal, Carbohydrates: 25 g, Protein: 6 g, Fat: 7 g, Fiber: 6 g

HEALTH BENEFITS:
Seasonal Produce Swap: Add spinach or kale for extra greens.
Dietary Substitutions: Replace chickpeas with white beans for a variation.

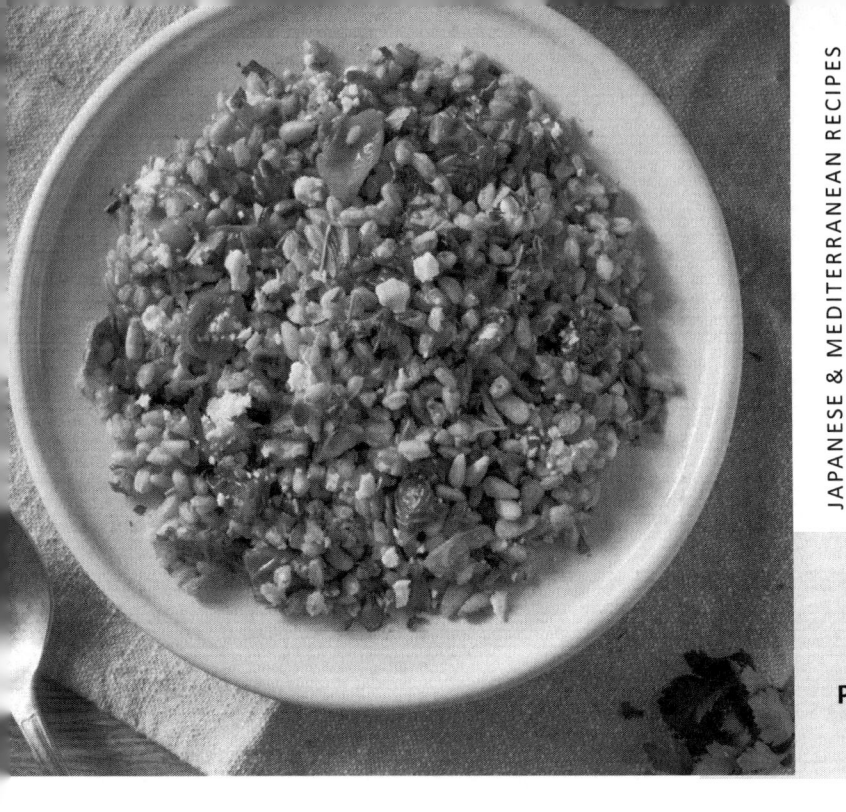

MEDITERRANEAN FARRO SALAD

Anti-Inflammatory Benefits:
Farro is rich in fiber and minerals, while vegetables like tomatoes and cucumbers provide antioxidants that keep up immune health and reduce inflammation.

PREP TIME: 10 MINS
COOK TIME: 20 MINS
SERVING: 4
Portion Size: 1 bowl per serving

INGREDIENTS

- 1 cup (200 g) farro, cooked according to the mentioned steps on the package instructions
- 1 cup (150 g) diced tomatoes
- 1/2 cup (75 g) diced cucumbers
- 1/4 cup (30 g) crumbled feta cheese
- 1/4 cup (10 g) fresh parsley, chopped
- 2 tbsp (30 ml) olive oil
- 1 tbsp (15 ml) lemon juice
- Salt and pepper to taste

EQUIPMENT NEEDED:
Saucepan, mixing bowl

INSTRUCTIONS

1. Take a large, deep-bottom bowl and combine cooked farro, tomatoes, cucumbers, feta cheese, and parsley.
2. Drizzle two tbsp oil and lemon juice, and powder it with salt and crushed pepper.
3. Toss softly to combine and serve immediately.

NUTRITIONAL INFORMATION (PER SERVING):

Calories: 220 kcal, Carbohydrates: 32 g, Protein: 6 g, Fat: 8 g, Fiber: 5 g

HEALTH BENEFITS:
Seasonal Produce Swap: Add roasted bell peppers or artichokes for variety.
Dietary Substitutions: Replace feta with dairy-free cheese for a vegan option.

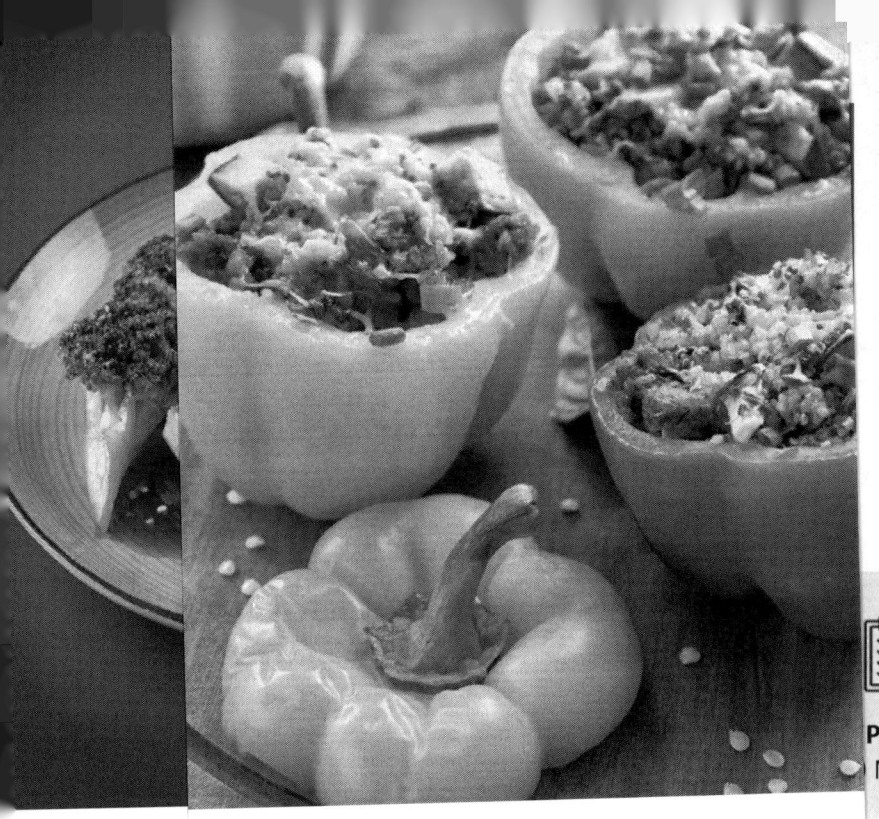

TOFU AND VEGETABLE SOBA NOODLES

Anti-Inflammatory Benefits:
Soba noodles are made from buckwheat, which contains anti-inflammatory properties, and tofu is a plant-based protein rich in essential nutrients.

PREP TIME: MINS **COOK TIME:** 15 MINS **SERVING: 3**
Portion Size: 1 bowl per serving

INGREDIENTS

- 3 large bell peppers (450 g), halved and seedless
- 1 cup (150 g) cooked quinoa
- 1/2 cup (75 g) diced tomatoes
- 1/4 cup (30 g) crumbled feta cheese
- 1/4 cup (10 g) fresh parsley, chopped
- 1 tbsp (15 ml) olive oil
- Salt and pepper to taste

INSTRUCTIONS

1. ...es according to the mentioned steps in the package ...n and set aside.
2. ...same oil in a skillet over moderate stove flame. Add ...sear for 5 minutes; keep stirring occasionally until
3. ...nd grated ginger, cooking for another 5 minutes until
4. ...auce and soba noodles, tossing to combine. Serve

INFORMATION (PER SERVING):
Ca...
...bohydrates: 30 g, Protein: 10 g, Fat: 7 g, Fiber: 4 g

Swap: Use asparagus or snap peas in spring.
Replace soba noodles with zucchini noodles for a

EQUIPMENT NEEDED:
Baking dish, saucepan

107

30-MINUTE MEALS

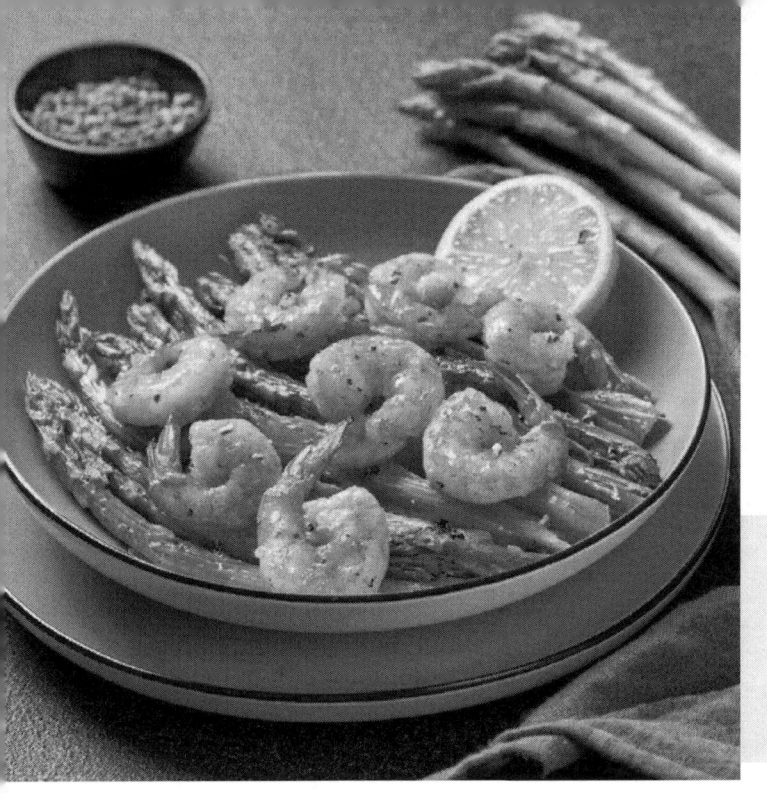

LEMON GARLIC SHRIMP WITH ASPARAGUS

30-MINUTE MEALS

Anti-Inflammatory Benefits:
Shrimp is a low-calorie protein source, while asparagus is rich in antioxidants and vitamins to combat inflammation.

PREP TIME: 5 MINS

COOK TIME: 10 MINS

SERVING: 2
Portion Size: 1 bowl per serving

INGREDIENTS

- 200 g shrimp, peeled and deveined
- 1 cup (150 g) asparagus, trimmed and cut into 2-inch pieces
- 2 cloves garlic, minced
- 1 tbsp (15 ml) olive oil
- 1 tbsp (15 ml) lemon juice
- Salt and pepper to taste

EQUIPMENT NEEDED:
Skillet, spatula

INSTRUCTIONS

1. Heat one tbsp oil in a skillet over moderate stove flame. Add garlic and sauté for 1 minute until fragrant.
2. Add shrimp and asparagus to the skillet. Cook for 5–7 minutes, keep stirring occasionally, until the shrimp is pink and cooked through.
3. Drizzle with lemon juice, powder it with salt and crushed pepper, and serve warm.

NUTRITIONAL INFORMATION (PER SERVING):

Calories: 180 kcal, Carbohydrates: 5 g, Protein: 20 g, Fat: 8 g, Fiber: 2 g

HEALTH BENEFITS:
Seasonal Produce Swap: Use snap peas or green beans instead of asparagus.
Dietary Substitutions: Replace shrimp with chicken or tofu for variety.

30-MINUTE MEALS

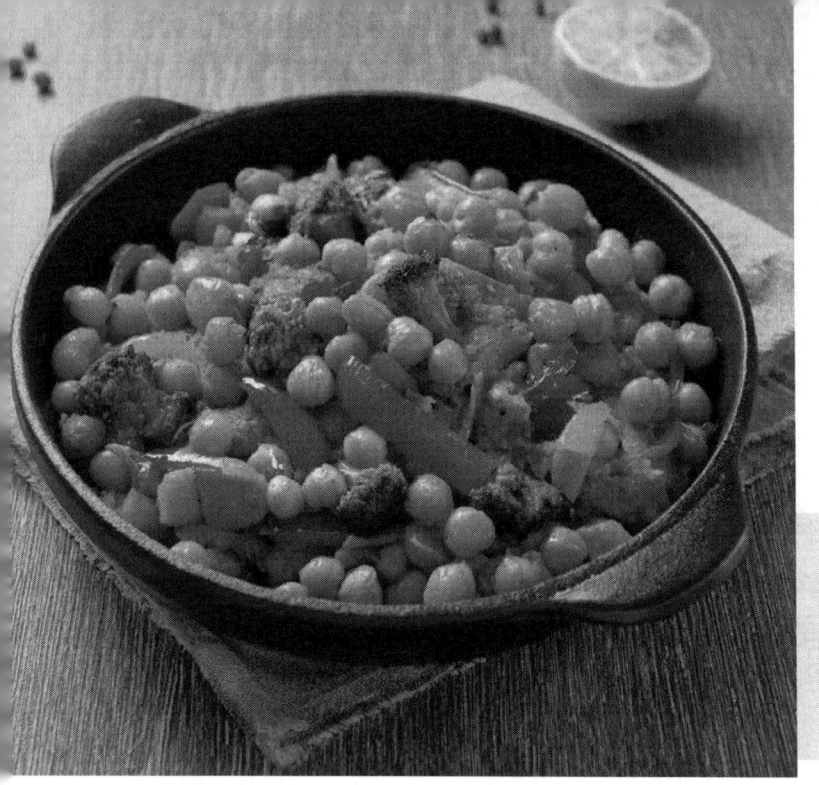

TURMERIC-SPICED CHICKPEA AND PEPPER STIR-FRY

Anti-Inflammatory Benefits:
Chickpeas provide plant-based protein and fiber, while turmeric offers potent anti-inflammatory and antioxidant properties.

PREP TIME: 5 MINS

COOK TIME: 10 MINS

SERVING: 2
Portion Size: 1 bowl per serving

INGREDIENTS

- 1 cup (150 g) cooked chickpeas
- 1/2 cup (50 g) sliced red bell pepper
- 1/2 cup (50 g) sliced yellow bell pepper
- 1/4 tsp (0.5 g) ground turmeric
- 1 tbsp (15 ml) olive oil
- Salt and pepper to taste

EQUIPMENT NEEDED:
Baking dish, pot, skillet

INSTRUCTIONS

1. Heat one tbsp oil in a skillet over moderate stove flame. Add bell peppers and sauté for 3–4 minutes until slightly softened.
2. Toss in the chickpeas, turmeric, salt, and pepper. Cook for more 5 minutes, stirring occasionally, until heated through.
3. Serve immediately with over rice or quinoa.

NUTRITIONAL INFORMATION (PER SERVING):

Calories: 150 kcal, Carbohydrates: 20 g, Protein: 6 g, Fat: 5 g, Fiber: 6 g

HEALTH BENEFITS:
Seasonal Produce Swap: Add zucchini or cherry tomatoes in summer.
Dietary Substitutions: Use black beans or lentils instead of chickpeas for variety.

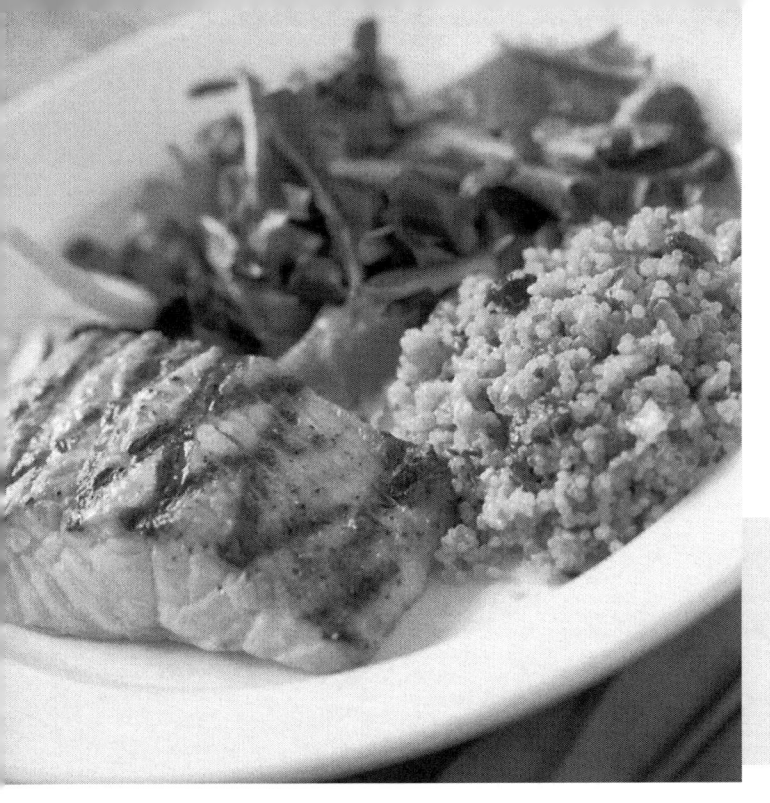

QUICK GRILLED SALMON WITH QUINOA

30-MINUTE MEALS

Anti-Inflammatory Benefits:
Salmon is high in omega-3 fatty acids, which reduce inflammation, while quinoa is a complete protein rich in essential amino acids.

PREP TIME: 5 MINS
COOK TIME: 15 MINS
SERVING: 2 Portion Size: 1 fillet and quinoa per serving

INGREDIENTS

- 2 salmon fillets (300 g total)
- 1/2 cup (90 g) quinoa
- 1 cup (240 ml) water
- 1 tbsp (15 ml) olive oil
- 1 tsp (2 g) garlic powder
- Salt and pepper to taste

EQUIPMENT NEEDED:
Grill or grill pan, saucepan

INSTRUCTIONS

1. Preheat grill or grill pan over moderate stove flame. Brush the fish fillets with one tbsp oil and powder it with garlic powder, salt, and pepper.
2. Grill the salmon for 4–5 minutes per side until cooked thoroughly.
3. While grilling, cook the quinoa in a saucepan with water according to the mentioned steps in the package instructions.
4. Serve the grilled salmon over the cooked quinoa.

NUTRITIONAL INFORMATION (PER SERVING):

Calories: 290 kcal, Carbohydrates: 12 g, Protein: 25 g, Fat: 15 g, Fiber: 3 g

HEALTH BENEFITS:
Seasonal Produce Swap: Add a side of steamed asparagus or roasted Brussels sprouts.
Dietary Substitutions: Use tofu or tempeh instead of salmon for a vegan option.

30-MINUTE MEALS

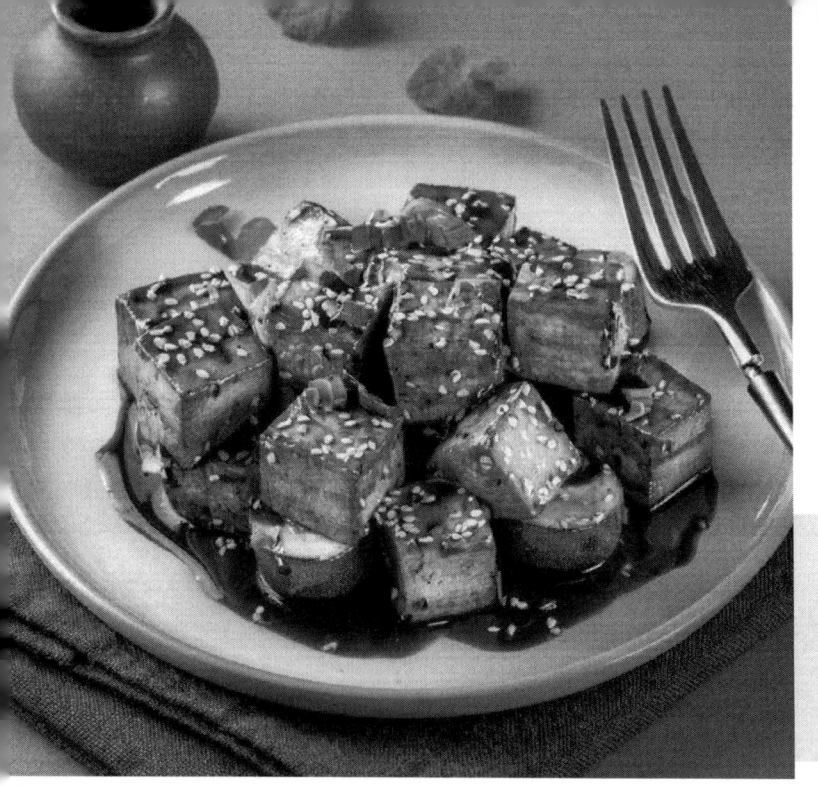

BALSAMIC GLAZED TOFU WITH ZUCCHINI

Anti-Inflammatory Benefits:
Tofu provides plant-based protein, while balsamic vinegar and zucchini add antioxidants and anti-inflammatory benefits.

PREP TIME: 5 MINS

COOK TIME: 10 MINS

SERVING: 2
Portion Size: 1 bowl per serving

INGREDIENTS

- 1 cup (150 g) firm tofu, cubed
- 1 cup (100 g) diced zucchini
- 2 tbsp (30 ml) balsamic vinegar
- 1 tbsp (15 ml) olive oil
- 1 tsp (5 ml) honey or maple syrup
- Salt and pepper to taste

EQUIPMENT NEEDED:
Skillet, spatula

INSTRUCTIONS

1. Heat one tbsp oil in a skillet over moderate stove flame. Add tofu and cook for 4–5 minutes, turning occasionally, until golden brown.
2. Add zucchini and cook for more 3–4 minutes until tender.
3. Drizzle with balsamic vinegar and sweetener (honey or maple syrup), stirring to coat. Cook for 1 minute, then powder it with salt and crushed pepper.
4. Serve warm as a main dish or over rice.

NUTRITIONAL INFORMATION (PER SERVING):

Calories: 180 kcal, Carbohydrates: 10 g, Protein: 10 g, Fat: 12 g, Fiber: 2 g

HEALTH BENEFITS:
Seasonal Produce Swap: Use summer squash or eggplant instead of zucchini.
Dietary Substitutions: Replace tofu with tempeh for a firmer texture.

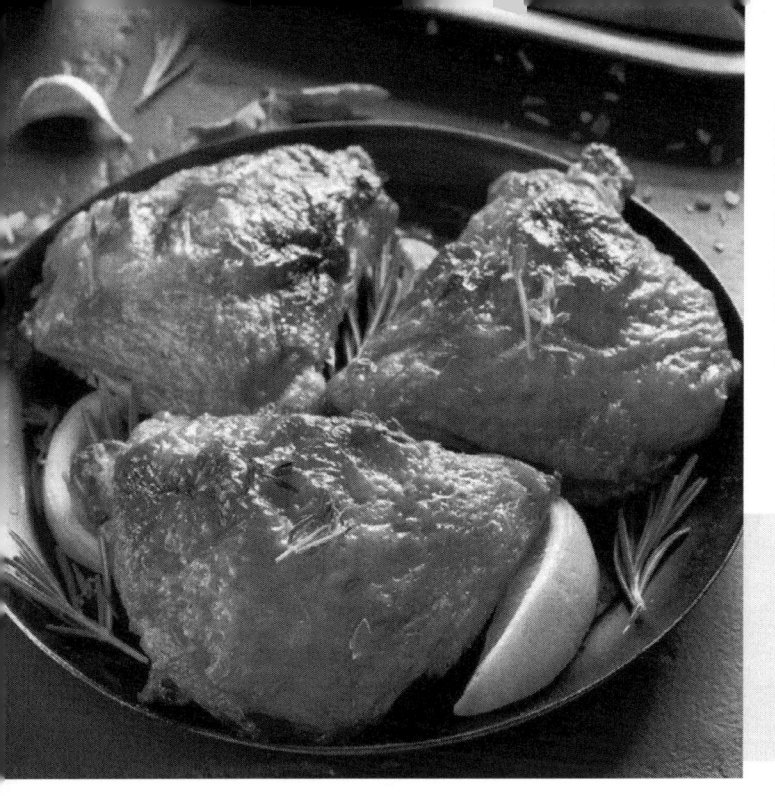

GARLIC LEMON CHICKEN THIGHS

30-MINUTE MEALS

Anti-Inflammatory Benefits:
Chicken thighs provide lean protein, while garlic and lemon offer antioxidants and immune-boosting properties.

PREP TIME: 5 MINS
COOK TIME: 20 MINS
SERVING: 3
Portion Size: 1 chicken thigh per serving

INGREDIENTS

- 3 chicken thighs (450 g), bone-in and skinless
- 2 cloves garlic, minced
- 1 tbsp (15 ml) olive oil
- 2 tbsp (30 ml) lemon juice
- 1 tsp (2 g) dried thyme
- Salt and pepper to taste

INSTRUCTIONS

1. Heat one tbsp oil in a skillet over moderate stove flame. Add thigh meat and cook for 5–7 minutes on one side until golden brown and cooked through.
2. Add mashed garlic and cook for 1 minute until fragrant.
3. Drizzle with lemon juice and sprinkle with thyme, cooking for an additional 2 minutes.
4. Powder it with salt and crushed pepper, then serve warm.

EQUIPMENT NEEDED:
Skillet, spatula

NUTRITIONAL INFORMATION (PER SERVING):

Calories: 200 kcal, Carbohydrates: 2 g, Protein: 25 g, Fat: 10 g, Fiber: 0 g

HEALTH BENEFITS:
Seasonal Produce Swap: Add roasted asparagus or green beans as a side.
Dietary Substitutions: Use tofu or tempeh as a plant-based alternative.

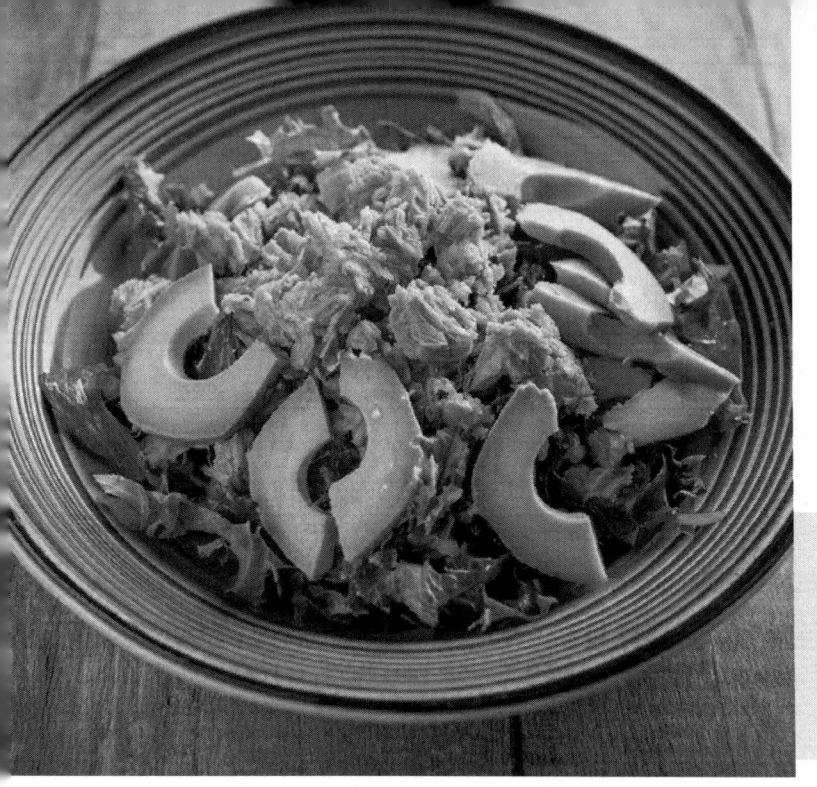

QUICK TUNA AND AVOCADO SALAD

30-MINUTE MEALS

Anti-Inflammatory Benefits:
Tuna is rich in omega-3 fatty acids, while avocado provides healthy fats and vitamins to reduce inflammation.

PREP TIME: 10 MINS
COOK TIME: 00 MINS
SERVING: 2
Portion Size: 1 bowl per serving

INGREDIENTS

- 1 can (120 g) tuna in water, drained
- 1 avocado (150 g), diced
- 1/4 cup (10 g) fresh parsley, chopped
- 1 tbsp (15 ml) olive oil
- 1 tbsp (15 ml) lemon juice
- Salt and pepper to taste

EQUIPMENT NEEDED:
Mixing bowl, fork

INSTRUCTIONS

1. Take a large, deep-bottom bowl and combine tuna, avocado, and parsley.
2. Drizzle one tbsp oil and lemon juice, and powder it with salt and crushed pepper.
3. Gently mix with a fork and serve immediately as a salad or sandwich filling.

NUTRITIONAL INFORMATION (PER SERVING):

Calories: 250 kcal, Carbohydrates: 5 g, Protein: 22 g, Fat: 15 g, Fiber: 4 g

HEALTH BENEFITS:

Seasonal Produce Swap: Add diced cucumber or cherry tomatoes for extra crunch.
Dietary Substitutions: Use chickpeas instead of tuna for a vegetarian option.

30-MINUTE MEALS

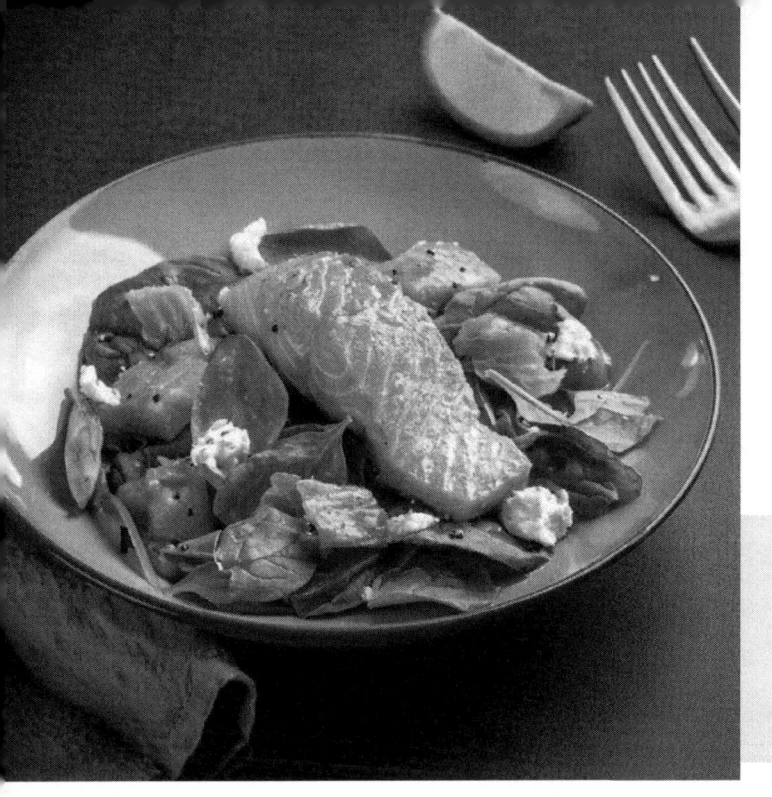

EASY SALMON AND SPINACH SALAD

Anti-Inflammatory Benefits:
Salmon provides omega-3 fatty acids, while spinach is packed with antioxidants and anti-inflammatory nutrients like vitamin K.

PREP TIME: 10 MINS

COOK TIME: 10 MINS

SERVING: 2
Portion Size: 1 salad per serving

INGREDIENTS

- 2 salmon fillets (300 g total)
- 4 cups (120 g) fresh spinach leaves
- 1/4 cup (40 g) cherry tomatoes, halved
- 2 tbsp (30 ml) olive oil
- 1 tbsp (15 ml) balsamic vinegar
- Salt and pepper to taste

EQUIPMENT NEEDED:
Skillet mixing bowl

INSTRUCTIONS

1. Heat 1 tbsp oil in a skillet. Cook salmon fillets for 4–5 minutes per side until cooked through.
2. Take a large deep-bottom bowl and combine spinach, cherry tomatoes, and 1 tbsp olive oil. Toss to coat.
3. Top the salad with the prepared salmon, then drizzle with balsamic vinegar.
4. Powder it with salt and crushed pepper, then serve warm or chilled.

NUTRITIONAL INFORMATION (PER SERVING):

Calories: 270 kcal, Carbohydrates: 8 g, Protein: 28 g, Fat: 14 g, Fiber: 3 g

HEALTH BENEFITS:
Seasonal Produce Swap: Add strawberries or blueberries for a summer twist.
Dietary Substitutions: Use tofu instead of salmon for a vegan option.

30-MINUTE MEALS

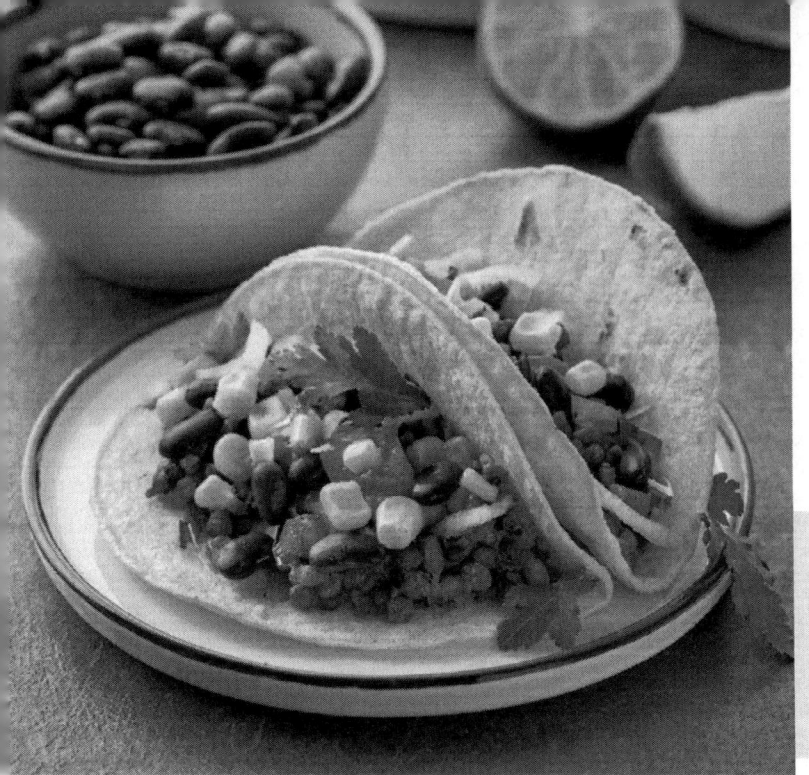

BLACK BEAN AND CORN TACOS

Anti-Inflammatory Benefits:
Black beans provide plant-based protein and fiber, while corn adds essential vitamins and minerals to combat inflammation.

PREP TIME: 10 MINS

COOK TIME: 10 MINS

SERVING: 4
Portion Size: 2 tacos per serving

INGREDIENTS

- 1 cup (150 g) cooked black beans
- 1/2 cup (75 g) corn kernels (fresh)
- 4 small corn tortillas
- 1/4 cup (40 g) diced red onion
- 1 tbsp (15 ml) lime juice
- 1 tbsp (15 ml) olive oil
- Salt and pepper to taste

EQUIPMENT NEEDED:
Skillet mixing bowl

INSTRUCTIONS

1. Heat one tbsp oil in a skillet over moderate stove flame. Add black beans with corn, and cook for 5 minutes until heated through.
2. Warm the tortillas
3. . Fill each tortilla with the black bean and corn mixture. Top with diced red onion and drizzle with lime juice.
4. Serve immediately.

NUTRITIONAL INFORMATION (PER SERVING):

Calories: 210 kcal, Carbohydrates: 30 g, Protein: 8 g, Fat: 6 g, Fiber: 6 g

HEALTH BENEFITS:
Seasonal Produce Swap: Add diced avocado or fresh salsa for extra flavor.
Dietary Substitutions: Use lettuce wraps instead of tortillas for a low-carb option.

ONE-POT DISHES

ONE-POT DISHES

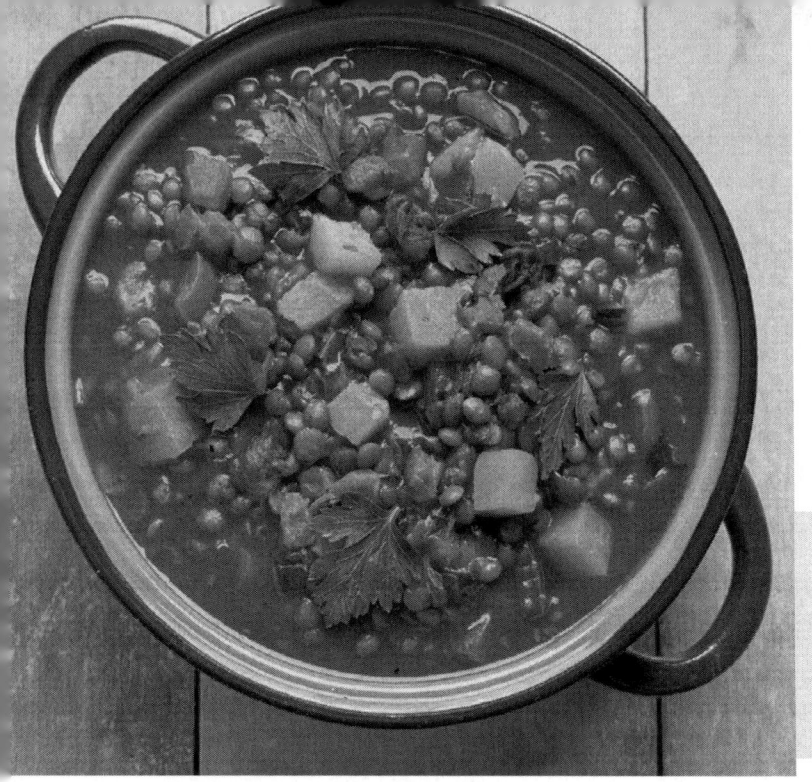

ONE-POT LENTIL AND VEGETABLE STEW

Anti-Inflammatory Benefits:
Lentils provide plant-based protein and fiber, while vegetables like carrots and celery are rich in antioxidants that help reduce inflammation.

PREP TIME: 10 MINS

COOK TIME: 25 MINS

SERVING: 4
Portion Size: 1 bowl per serving

INGREDIENTS

- 1 cup (200 g) cooked lentils
- 1 cup (100 g) diced carrots
- 1/2 cup (50 g) diced celery
- 1/2 cup (50 g) diced tomatoes
- 3 cups (720 ml) vegetable broth
- 1 tsp (2 g) ground cumin
- 1 tbsp (15 ml) olive oil
- Salt and pepper to taste

EQUIPMENT NEEDED:
Large pot, spoon

INSTRUCTIONS

1. Heat one tbsp oil in a pot over moderate stove flame. Add carrots and celery, and sauté for 5 minutes.
2. Toss in the lentils, tomatoes, vegetable broth, cumin, salt, and pepper.
3. Get it to a boil, then decrease the stove heat and simmer for 20 minutes, stirring occasionally.
4. Serve warm, garnished with fresh parsley.

NUTRITIONAL INFORMATION (PER SERVING):

Calories: 180 kcal, Carbohydrates: 25 g, Protein: 8 g, Fat: 4 g, Fiber: 7 g

HEALTH BENEFITS:
Seasonal Produce Swap: Add zucchini or green beans in summer.
Dietary Substitutions: Use chickpeas instead of lentils for variety.

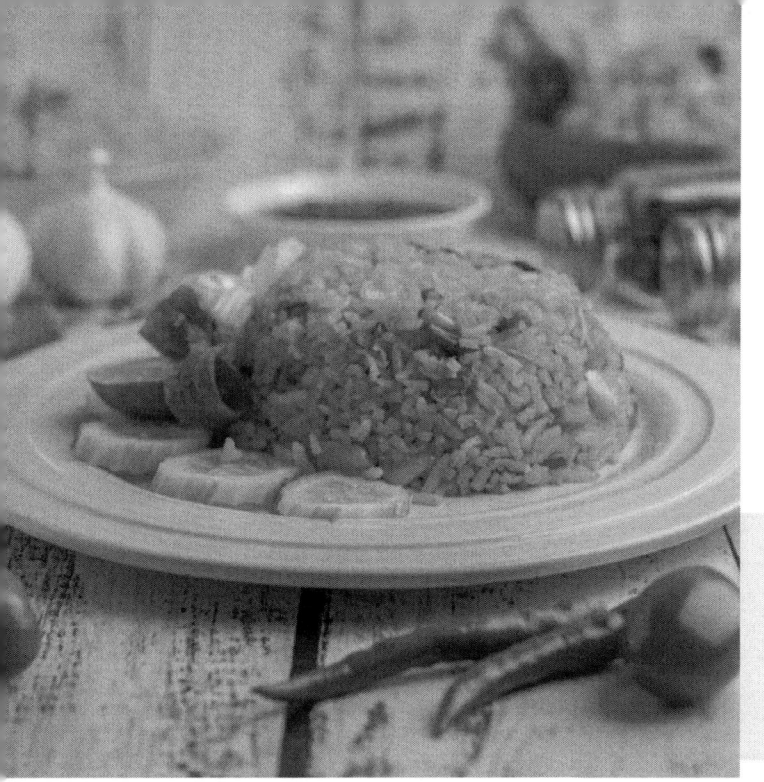

ONE-POT TURMERIC RICE WITH VEGGIES

ONE-POT DISHES

Anti-Inflammatory Benefits:
Turmeric provides curcumin, a potent anti-inflammatory compound, while rice and vegetables add essential nutrients and fiber.

PREP TIME: 10 MINS

COOK TIME: 20 MINS

SERVING: 3
Portion Size: 1 bowl per serving

INGREDIENTS

- 1 cup (180 g) long-grain rice
- 1/2 cup (50 g) diced carrots
- 1/2 cup (50 g) green peas
- 1/2 tsp (1 g) ground turmeric
- 2 cups (480 ml) vegetable broth
- 1 tbsp (15 ml) olive oil
- Salt and pepper to taste

INSTRUCTIONS

1. Heat one tbsp oil in a pot over moderate stove flame. Add rice and turmeric, stirring for 1 minute until the rice is lightly toasted.
2. Toss in the carrots, peas, and vegetable broth. Get it to a boil, then decrease
3. the stove heat, cover, and simmer for 17–20 minutes until the rice gets tender and the liquid is absorbed.
4. Powder it with salt and crushed pepper, then serve warm.

EQUIPMENT NEEDED:
Large pot, spoon

NUTRITIONAL INFORMATION (PER SERVING):

Calories: 200 kcal, Carbohydrates: 38 g, Protein: 4 g, Fat: 3 g, Fiber: 3 g

HEALTH BENEFITS:
Seasonal Produce Swap: Use asparagus or snap peas in spring.
Dietary Substitutions: Replace rice with quinoa for added protein.

ONE-POT DISHES

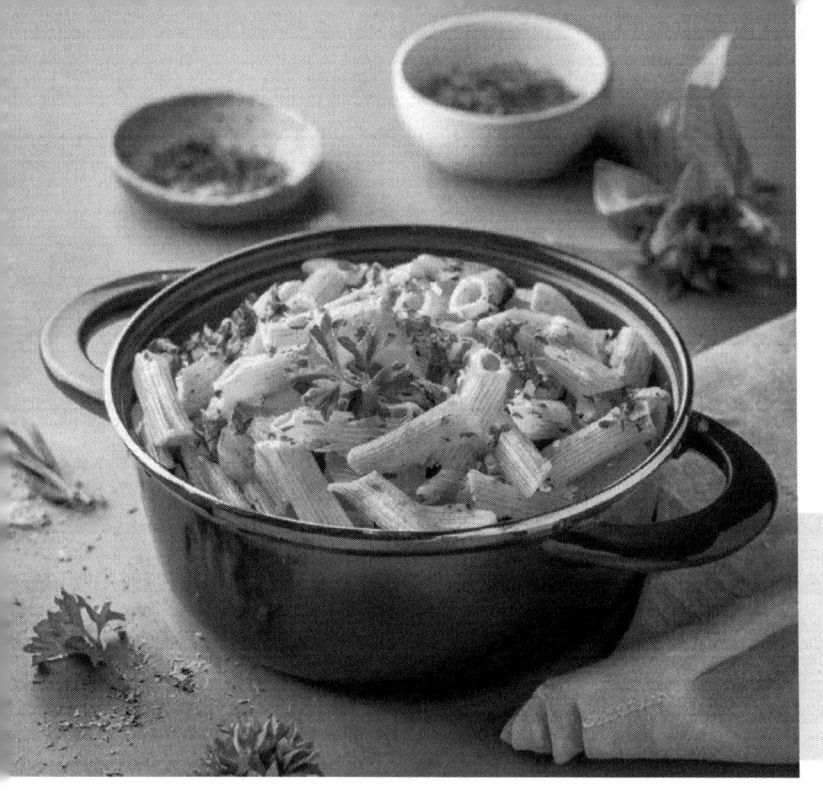

ONE-POT PASTA WITH FRESH HERBS

Anti-Inflammatory Benefits:
Whole-grain pasta is a good source of fiber, while fresh herbs like basil and parsley provide anti-inflammatory compounds and antioxidants.

PREP TIME: 5 MINS

COOK TIME: 15 MINS

SERVING: 3
Portion Size: 1 bowl per serving

INGREDIENTS

- 200 g whole-grain pasta
- 1 cup (150 g) cherry tomatoes, halved
- 1/2 cup (10 g) fresh basil, chopped
- 1/4 cup (10 g) fresh parsley, chopped
- 2 tbsp (30 ml) olive oil
- 2 cups (480 ml) vegetable broth
- Salt and pepper to taste

EQUIPMENT NEEDED:

Large pot, spoon

INSTRUCTIONS

1. In a pot, combine the pasta, cherry tomatoes, basil, parsley, olive oil, and vegetable broth.
2. Get it to a boil, then decrease the stove heat to medium and cook for 10–12 minutes, stirring occasionally, until the pasta is tender and most of the liquid is absorbed.
3. Powder it with salt and crushed pepper, and serve warm.

NUTRITIONAL INFORMATION (PER SERVING):

Calories: 250 kcal, Carbohydrates: 38 g, Protein: 7 g, Fat: 8 g, Fiber: 5 g

HEALTH BENEFITS:
Seasonal Produce Swap: Add zucchini or spinach for extra greens.
Dietary Substitutions: Use gluten-free pasta for a gluten-free option.

ONE-POT DISHES

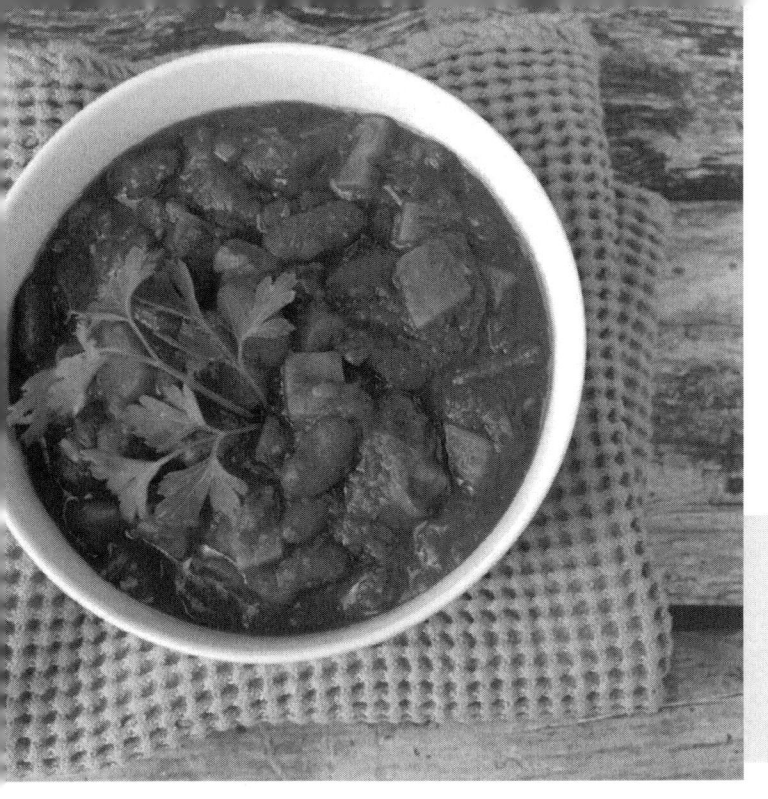

SWEET POTATO AND BLACK BEAN CHILI

Anti-Inflammatory Benefits:
Sweet potatoes are rich in beta-carotene, while black beans provide protein and fiber to support gut health and reduce inflammation.

PREP TIME: 10 MINS

COOK TIME: 20 MINS

SERVING: 4
Portion Size: 1 bowl per serving

INGREDIENTS

- 1 cup (150 g) cooked black beans
- 1 cup (150 g) diced sweet potatoes
- 1/2 cup (50 g) diced red bell peppers
- 2 cups (480 ml) vegetable broth
- 1 tsp (2 g) ground cumin
- 1/2 tsp (1 g) chili powder
- 1 tbsp (15 ml) olive oil
- Salt and pepper to taste

INSTRUCTIONS

1. Heat one tbsp oil in a pot over moderate stove flame. Add sweet potatoes and red bell peppers, and sauté for 5 minutes.
2. Toss in the black beans, vegetable broth, cumin, chili powder, salt, and pepper.
3. Get it to a boil, then decrease the stove heat and simmer for 15 minutes until the sweet potatoes are tender.
4. Serve warm, garnished with fresh cilantro or avocado slices.

EQUIPMENT NEEDED:
Large pot, spoon

NUTRITIONAL INFORMATION (PER SERVING):

Calories: 200 kcal, Carbohydrates: 30 g, Protein: 8 g, Fat: 5 g, Fiber: 7 g

HEALTH BENEFITS:
Seasonal Produce Swap: Add diced zucchini or corn in summer.
Dietary Substitutions: Use kidney beans or chickpeas for variety.

ONE-POT DISHES

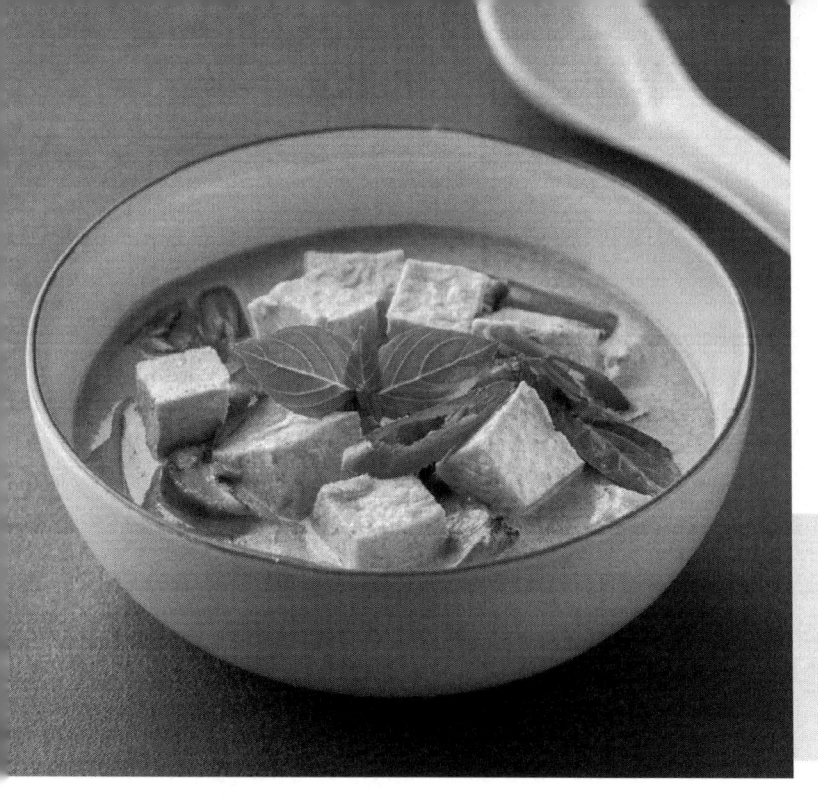

THAI GREEN CURRY WITH TOFU

Anti-Inflammatory Benefits:
Coconut milk contains healthy fats that reduce inflammation, while green curry paste includes anti-inflammatory spices like turmeric and ginger.

PREP TIME: 10 MINS

COOK TIME: 20 MINS

SERVING: 3
Portion Size: 1 bowl per serving

INGREDIENTS

- 1 cup (200 g) firm tofu, cubed
- 1 cup (100 g) diced zucchini
- 1/2 cup (50 g) sliced bell peppers
- 1 tbsp (15 ml) green curry paste
- 1 cup (240 ml) coconut milk
- 1 cup (240 ml) vegetable broth
- 1 tbsp (15 ml) olive oil
- 1 tsp (5 ml) lime juice

INSTRUCTIONS

1. Heat one tbsp oil in a pot over moderate stove flame. Add tofu and cook for 5 minutes until lightly browned.
2. Toss in the green curry paste and cook for 1 minute until fragrant.
3. Add zucchini, bell peppers, coconut milk, and vegetable broth. Get it to a boil, then decrease the stove heat and simmer for 15 minutes.
4. Toss in lime juice before serving.

EQUIPMENT NEEDED:
Pot, spoon

NUTRITIONAL INFORMATION (PER SERVING):

Calories: 200 kcal, Carbohydrates: 10 g, Protein: 8 g, Fat: 14 g, Fiber: 3 g

HEALTH BENEFITS:
Seasonal Produce Swap: Add snap peas or asparagus in spring.
Dietary Substitutions: Use tempeh instead of tofu for a firmer texture.

ONE-POT DISHES

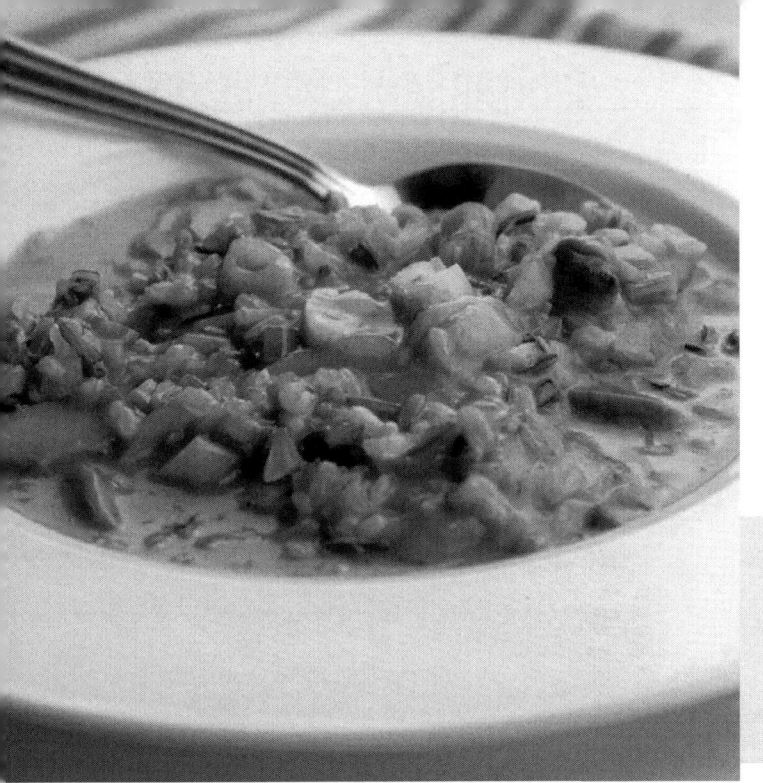

WILD RICE AND MUSHROOM SOUP

Anti-Inflammatory Benefits:
Wild rice is high in fiber and nutrients, while mushrooms contain anti-inflammatory compounds and support immune health.

PREP TIME: 10 MINS
COOK TIME: 30 MINS
SERVING: 4 Portion Size: 1 bowl per serving

INGREDIENTS

- 1 cup (150 g) cooked wild rice
- 1 cup (100 g) sliced mushrooms
- 1/2 cup (50 g) diced carrots
- 1/2 cup (50 g) diced celery
- 3 cups (720 ml) vegetable broth
- 1 tbsp (15 ml) olive oil
- Salt and pepper to taste

EQUIPMENT NEEDED:
Large pot, spoon

INSTRUCTIONS

1. Heat one tbsp oil in a pot over moderate stove flame. Add carrots, celery, and mushrooms, and sauté for 5 minutes.
2. Toss in the wild rice and vegetable broth. Get it to a boil, then decrease the stove heat and simmer for 20 minutes.
3. Powder it with salt and crushed pepper, then serve warm.

NUTRITIONAL INFORMATION (PER SERVING):

Calories: 170 kcal, Carbohydrates: 28 g, Protein: 5 g, Fat: 4 g, Fiber: 4 g

HEALTH BENEFITS:
Seasonal Produce Swap: Add spinach or kale for extra greens.
Dietary Substitutions: Replace wild rice with brown rice for a milder flavor.

ONE-POT DISHES

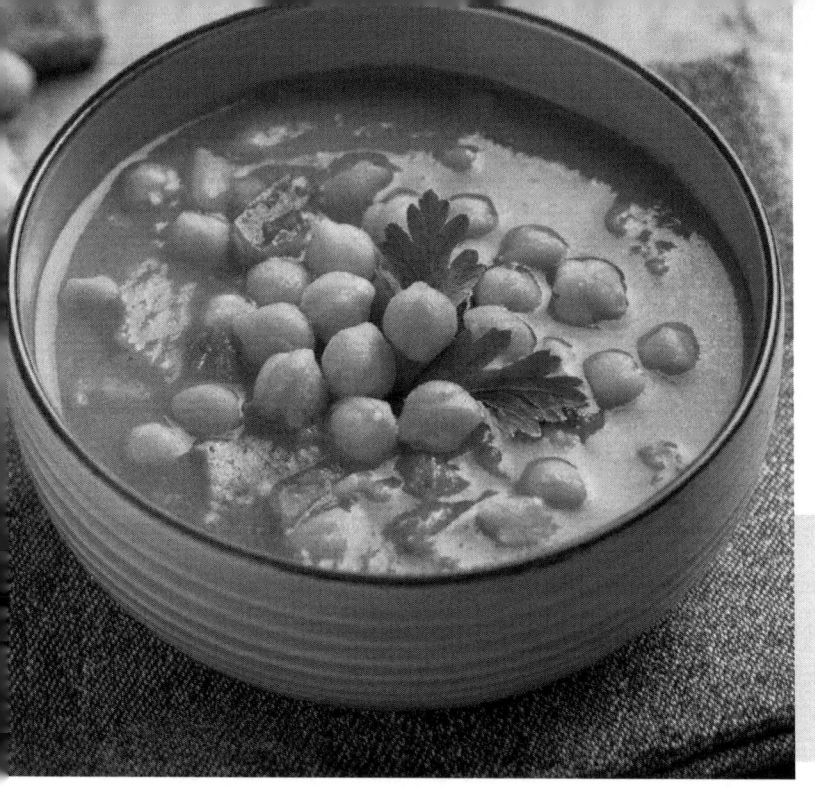

MEDITERRANEAN CHICKPEA SOUP

Anti-Inflammatory Benefits:
Chickpeas provide plant-based protein and fiber, while olive oil and tomatoes add heart-healthy antioxidants.

PREP TIME: 10 MINS

COOK TIME: 20 MINS

SERVING: 4
Portion Size: 1 bowl per serving

INGREDIENTS

- 1 cup (150 g) cooked chickpeas
- 1/2 cup (50 g) diced tomatoes
- 1/2 cup (50 g) diced onion
- 2 cups (480 ml) vegetable broth
- 1 tbsp (15 ml) olive oil
- 1/2 tsp (1 g) dried oregano
- Salt and pepper to taste

EQUIPMENT NEEDED:
Pot, spoon

INSTRUCTIONS

1. Heat one tbsp oil in a pot over moderate stove flame. Add onion and soften for 3 minutes.
2. Toss in the chickpeas, tomatoes, vegetable broth, oregano, salt, and pepper.
3. Get it to a boil, then decrease the stove heat and simmer for 15 minutes.
4. Serve warm with a side of whole-grain bread.

NUTRITIONAL INFORMATION (PER SERVING):

Calories: 190 kcal, Carbohydrates: 25 g, Protein: 8 g, Fat: 6 g, Fiber: 6 g

HEALTH BENEFITS:
Seasonal Produce Swap: Add diced zucchini or squash in summer.
Dietary Substitutions: Use cannellini beans instead of chickpeas for variety.

ONE-POT DISHES

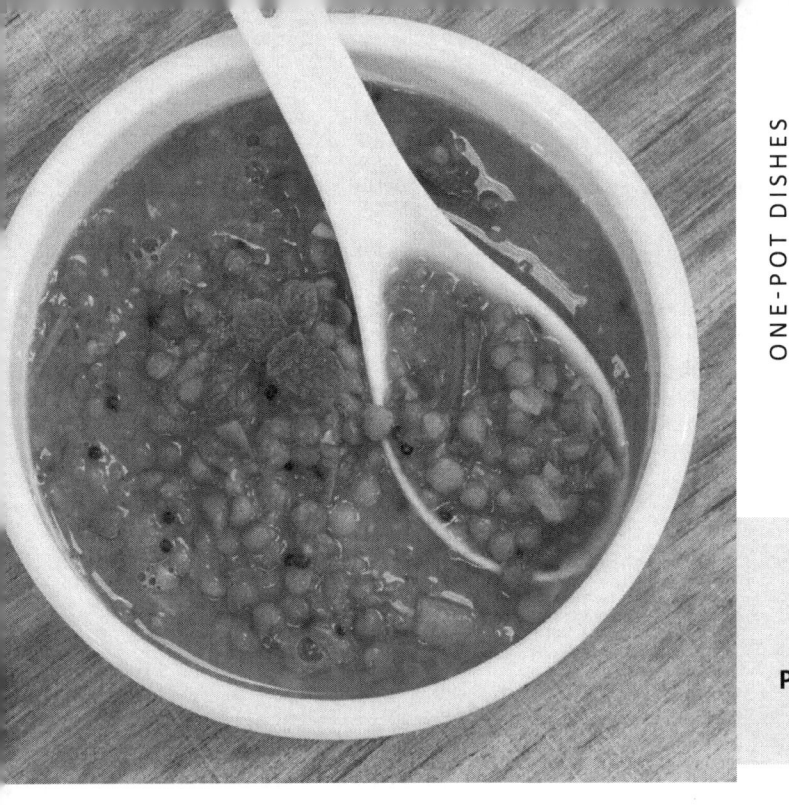

INDIAN-SPICED LENTIL STEW

Anti-Inflammatory Benefits:
Lentils are packed with fiber and plant-based protein, while spices like turmeric and cumin provide powerful anti-inflammatory effects.

PREP TIME: 10 MINS

COOK TIME: 25 MINS

SERVING: 4
Portion Size: 1 bowl per serving

INGREDIENTS

- 1 cup (200 g) cooked lentils
- 1/2 cup (50 g) diced onion
- 1/2 cup (50 g) diced tomatoes
- 1/2 cup (50 g) diced carrots
- 2 cups (480 ml) vegetable broth
- 1 tsp (2 g) ground turmeric
- 1 tsp (2 g) ground cumin
- 1 tbsp (15 ml) olive oil
- Salt and pepper to taste

EQUIPMENT NEEDED:
Large pot, spoon

INSTRUCTIONS

1. Heat one tbsp oil in a pot over moderate stove flame. Add onion and carrots, and sauté for 5 minutes.
2. Toss in lentils, tomatoes, vegetable broth, turmeric, cumin, salt, and pepper.
3. Get it to a boil, then decrease the stove heat and simmer for 20 minutes.
4. Serve warm, garnished with fresh cilantro or a dollop of yogurt.

NUTRITIONAL INFORMATION (PER SERVING):

Calories: 200 kcal, Carbohydrates: 28 g, Protein: 10 g, Fat: 5 g, Fiber: 8 g

HEALTH BENEFITS:
Seasonal Produce Swap: Add spinach or kale in winter for extra greens.
Dietary Substitutions: Use split peas instead of lentils for a different flavor.

SNACKS: SWEET & SAVORY

SNACKS: SWEET & SAVORY

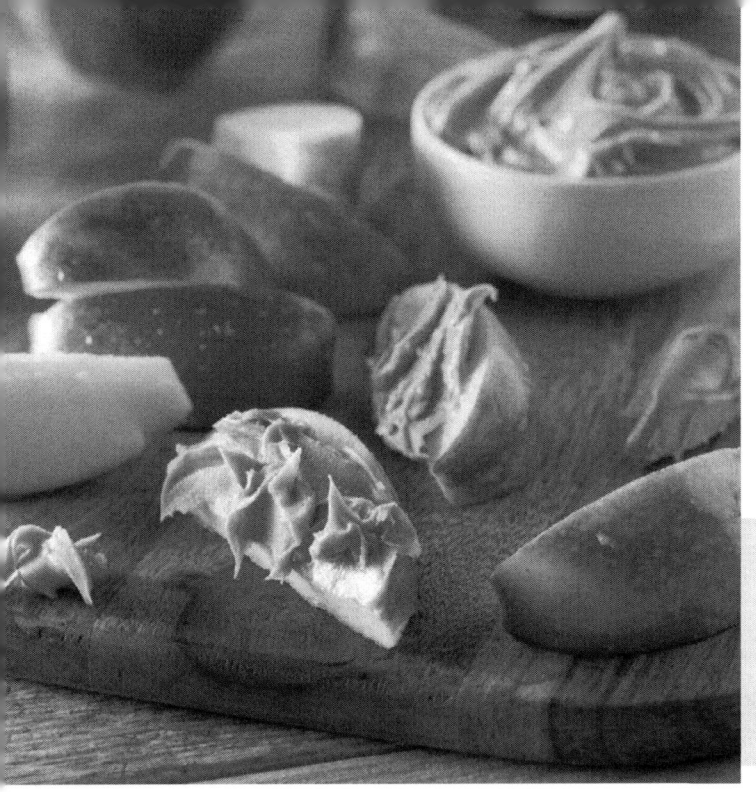

APPLE SLICES WITH ALMOND BUTTER

Anti-Inflammatory Benefits:
Apples are rich in antioxidants like quercetin, and almond butter provides healthy fats and vitamin E to reduce inflammation.

PREP TIME: 5 MINS

COOK TIME: 00 MINS

SERVING: 2
Portion Size: 1 apple with almond butter per serving

INGREDIENTS

- 1 medium apple (200 g), sliced
- 2 tbsp (30 g) almond butter

INSTRUCTIONS

1. Slice the apple into thin wedges.
2. Serve the apple slices with almond butter for dipping.

EQUIPMENT NEEDED:
Knife, spoon

NUTRITIONAL INFORMATION (PER SERVING):

Calories: 150 kcal, Carbohydrates: 18 g, Protein: 3 g, Fat: 8 g, Fiber: 4 g

HEALTH BENEFITS:
Seasonal Produce Swap: Use pears or peaches in place of apples.
Dietary Substitutions: Replace almond butter with sunflower seed butter for a nut-free option.

SNACKS: SWEET & SAVORY

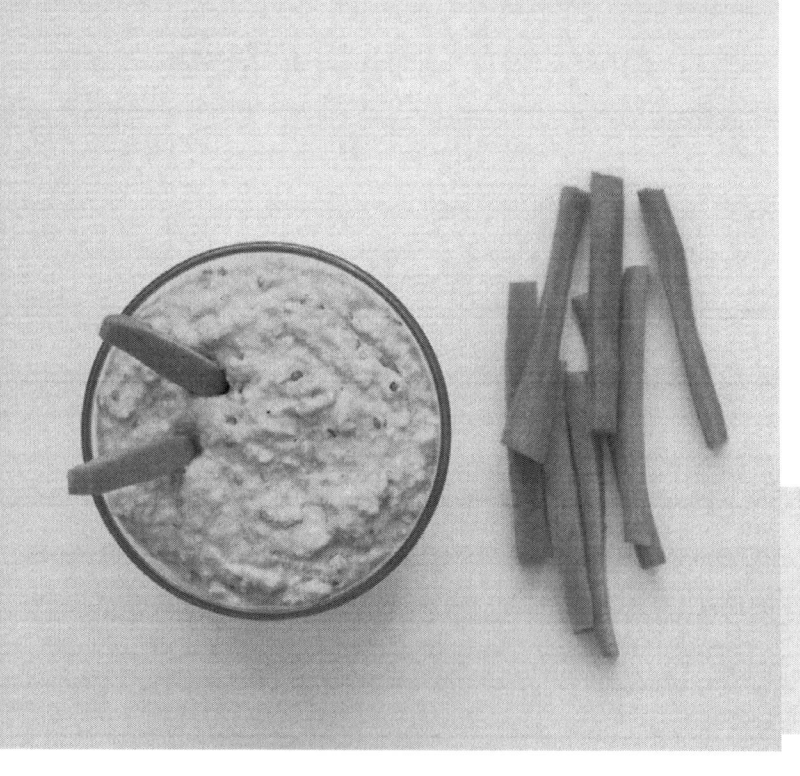

CARROT STICKS WITH HUMMUS

Anti-Inflammatory Benefits:
Carrots are a great source of beta-carotene, while hummus provides plant-based protein and heart-healthy fats.

PREP TIME: 5 MINS

COOK TIME: 00 MINS

SERVING: 2
Portion Size: 1/2 cup carrots with 2 tbsp hummus per serving

INGREDIENTS

- 1 cup (100 g) carrot sticks
- 4 tbsp (60 g) hummus

EQUIPMENT NEEDED:
Knife, small bowl

INSTRUCTIONS

1. Slice carrots into sticks or use pre-cut baby carrots.
2. Serve with hummus in a small bowl for dipping.

NUTRITIONAL INFORMATION (PER SERVING):

Calories: 120 kcal, Carbohydrates: 10 g, Protein: 3 g, Fat: 6 g, Fiber: 4 g

HEALTH BENEFITS:

Seasonal Produce Swap: Use cucumber sticks or bell pepper slices instead of carrots.
Dietary Substitutions: Use tahini sauce instead of hummus for a variation.

SNACKS: SWEET & SAVORY

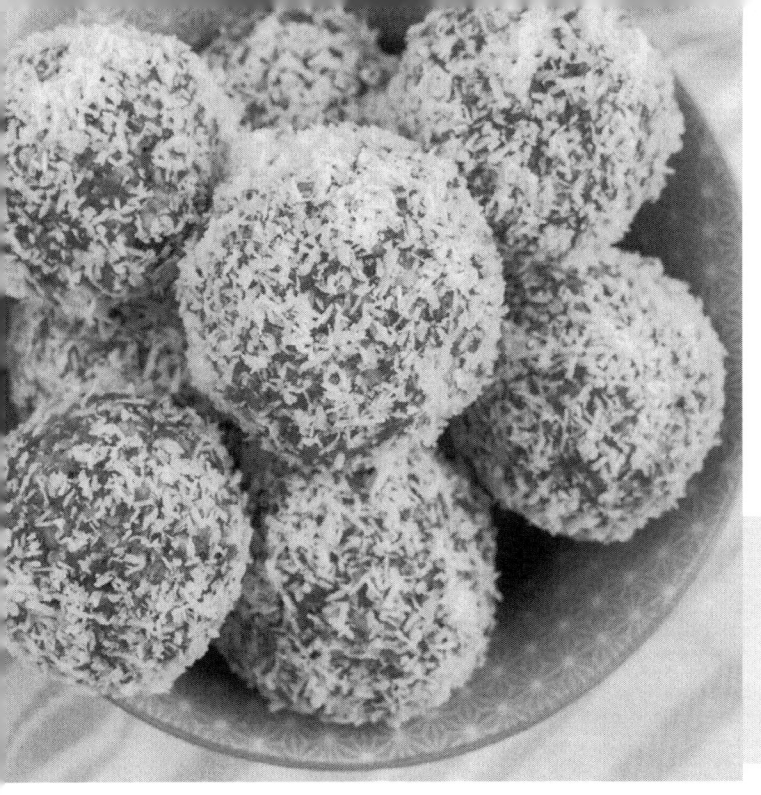

COCONUT AND ALMOND ENERGY BALLS

Anti-Inflammatory Benefits:
Coconut and almonds are rich in healthy fats, while dates provide natural sweetness and fiber to support digestion.

PREP TIME: 10 MINS

COOK TIME: 00 MINS

SERVING: 6
Portion Size: 3 energy balls per serving

INGREDIENTS

- 1/2 cup (50 g) almonds
- 1/4 cup (25 g) shredded unsweetened coconut
- 4 dates (80 g), pitted
- 1 tbsp (15 ml) coconut oil
- 1 tsp (5 ml) vanilla extract

EQUIPMENT NEEDED:
Food processor, small bowl

INSTRUCTIONS

1. In a food blender, blend the almonds with coconut until finely chopped.
2. Add dates with one tbsp coconut oil, and vanilla extract, and blend on full power until the mixture forms a sticky dough.
3. Roll the mixture into 6 small balls.
4. Chill for 15 minutes before serving.

NUTRITIONAL INFORMATION (PER SERVING):

Calories: 200 kcal, Carbohydrates: 15 g, Protein: 4 g, Fat: 14 g, Fiber: 4 g

HEALTH BENEFITS:
Seasonal Produce Swap: Add dried cranberries or apricots for extra flavor.
Dietary Substitutions: Use sunflower seeds instead of almonds for a nut-free option.

SNACKS: SWEET & SAVORY

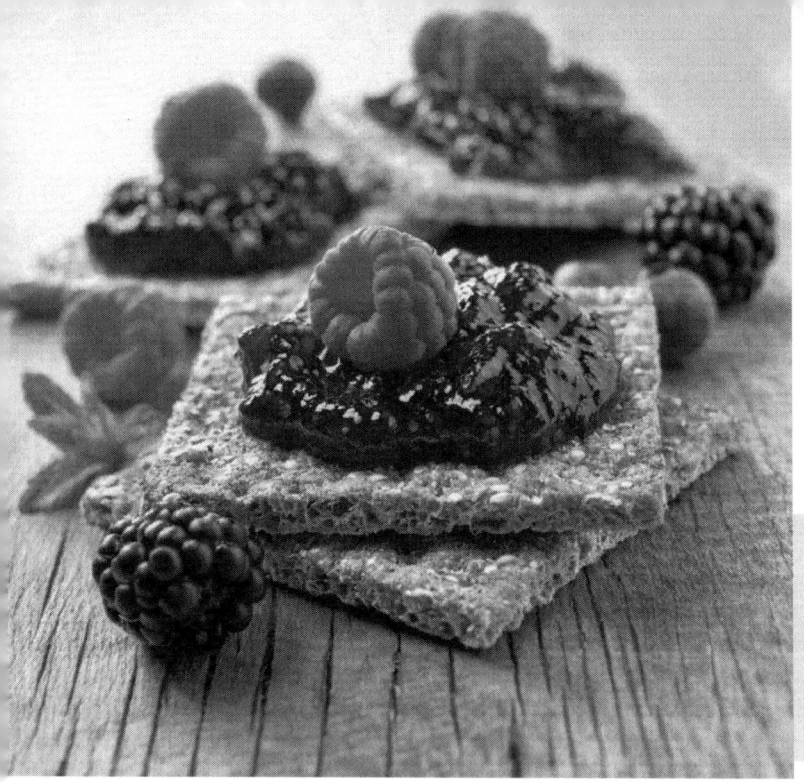

BERRY CHIA JAM ON WHOLE-GRAIN CRACKERS

Anti-Inflammatory Benefits:
Chia seeds are abundant in omega-3 fatty acids, and berries are rich in antioxidants to fight inflammation.

PREP TIME: 5 MINS

COOK TIME: 10 MINS

SERVING: 2
Portion Size: 3 crackers with jam per serving

INGREDIENTS

- 1/2 cup (75 g) fresh mixed berries
- 1 tbsp (15 g) chia seeds
- 6 whole-grain crackers

EQUIPMENT NEEDED:
Saucepan, spoon

INSTRUCTIONS

1. Heat berries in a small saucepan over moderate stove flame, stirring until they break down into a sauce (about 5 minutes).
2. Toss in chia seeds and cook for another 2–3 minutes until thickened. Let cool.
3. Spread the chia jam onto whole-grain crackers and serve immediately.

NUTRITIONAL INFORMATION (PER SERVING):

Calories: 150 kcal, Carbohydrates: 20 g, Protein: 3 g, Fat: 6 g, Fiber: 5 g

HEALTH BENEFITS:

Seasonal Produce Swap: Use strawberries, raspberries, or peaches based on availability.
Dietary Substitutions: Replace crackers with rice cakes for a gluten-free option.

SNACKS: SWEET & SAVORY

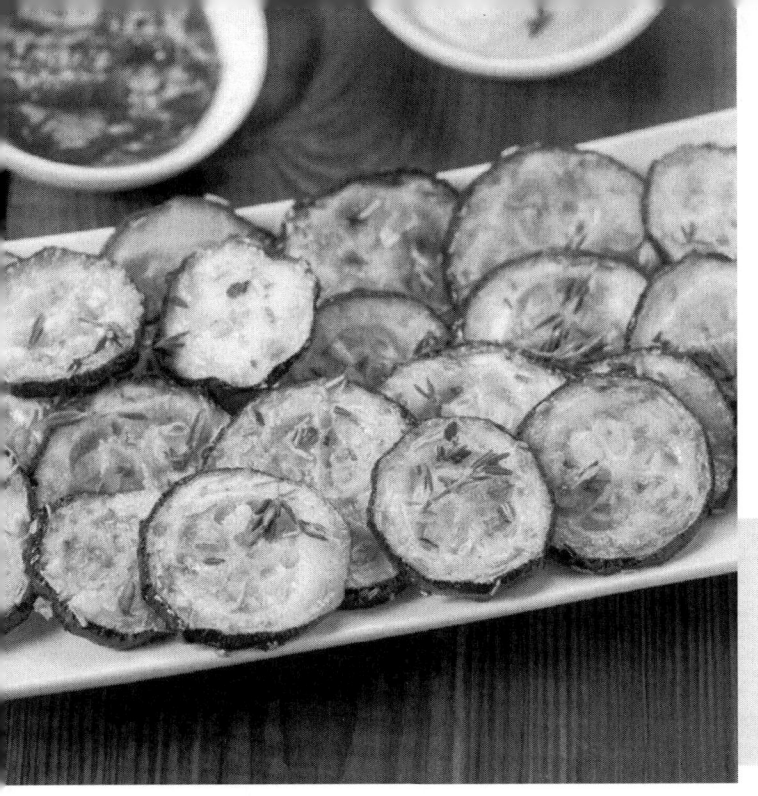

BAKED ZUCCHINI CHIPS

Anti-Inflammatory Benefits:
Zucchini is low in calories and high in antioxidants, making it a healthy, anti-inflammatory snack.

PREP TIME: 10 MINS
COOK TIME: 15 MINS
SERVING: 3
Portion Size: 1 cup per serving

INGREDIENTS

- 2 medium zucchinis (400 g), thinly sliced
- 1 tbsp (15 ml) olive oil
- 1/2 tsp (2 g) garlic powder
- 1/4 tsp (1 g) salt

INSTRUCTIONS

1. Preheat oven to 400°F (200°C). Arrange the baking sheet with parchment paper.
2. Toss zucchini slices with olive oil, garlic powder, and salt. Arrange in a single layer on the paper-arranged baking sheet.
3. Bake for 12–15 minutes, flipping halfway, until crispy and golden.
4. Let cool slightly before serving.

EQUIPMENT NEEDED:
Baking sheet, parchment paper

NUTRITIONAL INFORMATION (PER SERVING):

Calories: 80 kcal, Carbohydrates: 5 g, Protein: 1 g, Fat: 6 g, Fiber: 2 g

HEALTH BENEFITS:
Seasonal Produce Swap: Use sweet potatoes or eggplant for variation.
Dietary Substitutions: Add nutritional yeast for a cheesy flavor.

SNACKS: SWEET & SAVORY

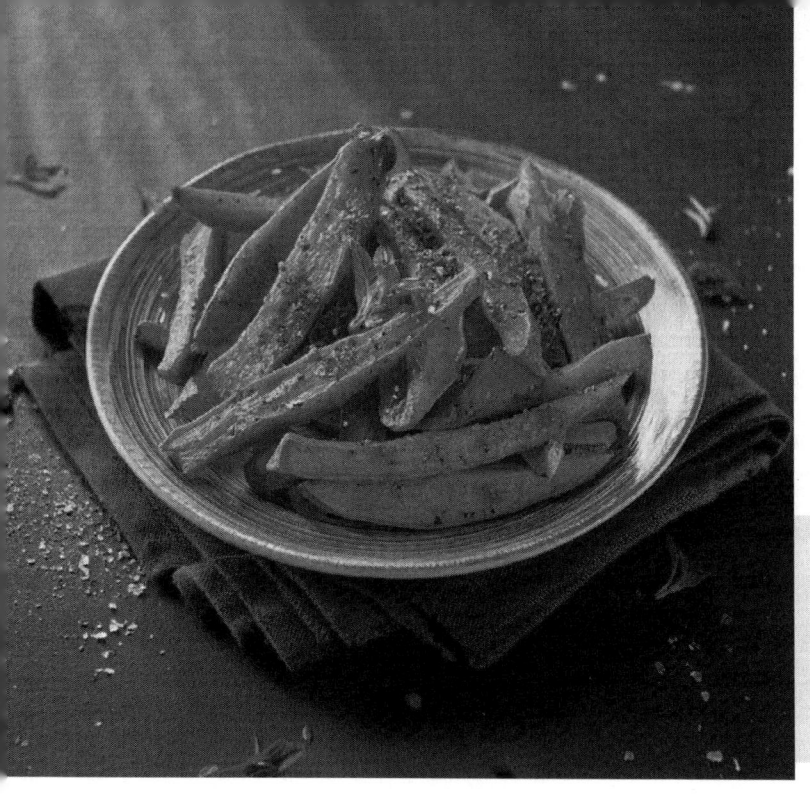

SWEET POTATO FRIES WITH PAPRIKA

Anti-Inflammatory Benefits:
Sweet potatoes are rich in beta-carotene and antioxidants, while paprika adds anti-inflammatory properties and enhances flavor.

PREP TIME: 10 MINS

COOK TIME: 20 MINS

SERVING: 3
Portion Size: 1 cup per serving

INGREDIENTS

- 2 medium sweet potatoes (400 g), cut into thin fries
- 1 tbsp (15 ml) olive oil
- 1 tsp (2 g) paprika
- 1/4 tsp (1 g) salt

EQUIPMENT NEEDED:
Baking sheet, parchment paper

INSTRUCTIONS

1. Preheat oven to 425°F (220°C). Arrange the baking sheet with parchment paper.
2. Toss the potato fries with one tbsp oil, paprika, and salt. Spread them out in a single layer on the paper-arranged baking sheet.
3. Bake for 17-20 minutes, flip after halftime has passed, until golden and crispy.
4. Let cool slightly and serve warm.

NUTRITIONAL INFORMATION (PER SERVING):

Calories: 130 kcal, Carbohydrates: 22 g, Protein: 2 g, Fat: 4 g, Fiber: 4 g

HEALTH BENEFITS:
Seasonal Produce Swap: Use carrots or parsnips for variation.
Dietary Substitutions: Add chili powder for a spicier option.

132

SNACKS: SWEET & SAVORY

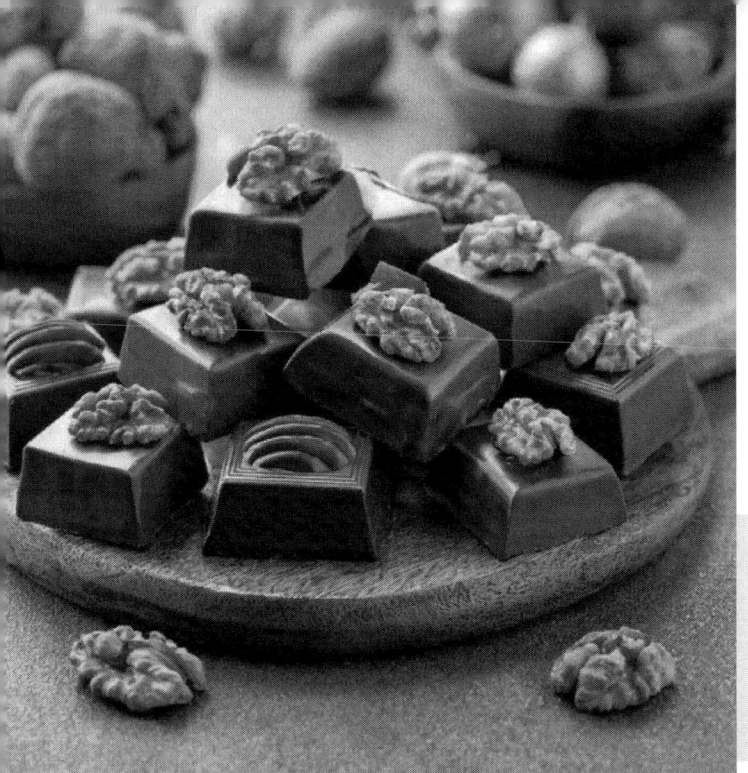

DARK CHOCOLATE AND WALNUT CLUSTERS

Anti-Inflammatory Benefits:
Dark chocolate is high in flavonoids, which are powerful antioxidants, while walnuts provide omega-3 fatty acids to reduce inflammation.

PREP TIME: 10 MINS

COOK TIME: 00 MINS

SERVING: 6
Portion Size: 3 clusters per serving

INGREDIENTS

- 1/2 cup (50 g) dark chocolate chips (70% or higher cocoa)
- 1/2 cup (50 g) walnut halves

INSTRUCTIONS

1. Melt the dark chocolate, keep stirring through this time until smooth.
2. Toss in walnut halves until evenly coated with chocolate.
3. Drop fully loaded spoonfuls of the mixture onto a sheet of parchment paper to form clusters.
4. Chill in the refrigerator for 15 minutes or until the chocolate is set. Serve chilled.

EQUIPMENT NEEDED:
Mixing bowl, parchment paper

NUTRITIONAL INFORMATION (PER SERVING):
Calories: 180 kcal, Carbohydrates: 10 g, Protein: 3 g, Fat: 15 g, Fiber: 2 g

HEALTH BENEFITS:
Seasonal Produce Swap: Add dried cranberries or coconut flakes for extra flavor.
Dietary Substitutions: Use dairy-free dark chocolate for a vegan option.

SNACKS: SWEET & SAVORY

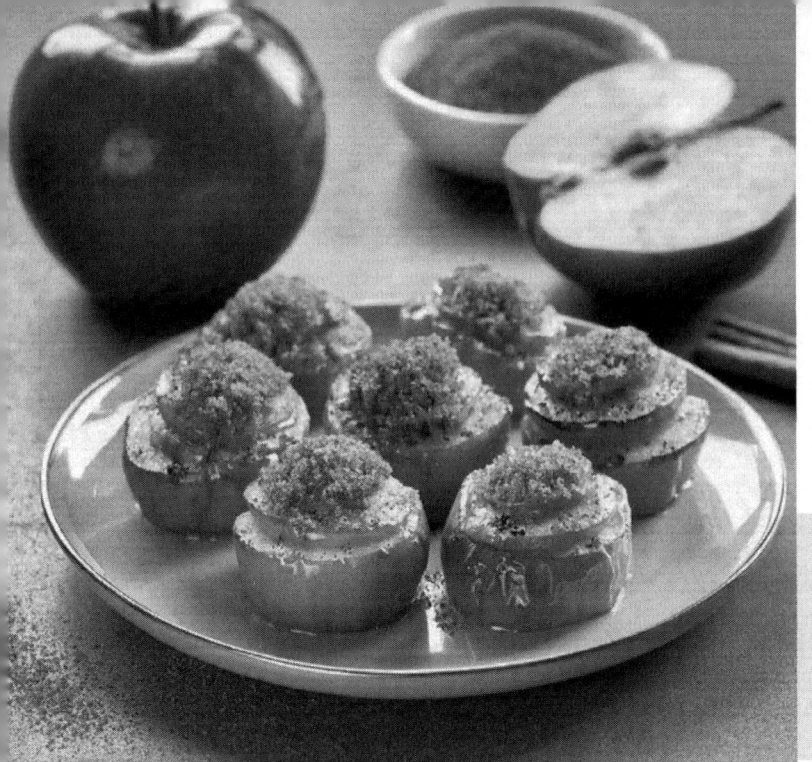

APPLE AND CINNAMON BITES

Anti-Inflammatory Benefits:
Apples are rich in antioxidants, while cinnamon has powerful anti-inflammatory and blood sugar-regulating properties.

PREP TIME: 5 MINS

COOK TIME: 00 MINS

SERVING: 2
Portion Size: 1 apple per serving

INGREDIENTS

- 2 medium apples (400 g total), sliced
- 1/2 tsp (1 g) ground cinnamon
- 1 tsp (5 ml) honey or maple syrup (optional)

EQUIPMENT NEEDED:
Knife, small bowl

INSTRUCTIONS

1. Arrange apple slices on a plate.
2. Sprinkle with cinnamon and drizzle sweetener (honey or maple syrup) if desired.
3. Serve immediately as a quick and healthy snack.

NUTRITIONAL INFORMATION (PER SERVING):

Calories: 100 kcal, Carbohydrates: 22 g, Protein: 0 g, Fat: 0 g, Fiber: 4 g

HEALTH BENEFITS:
Seasonal Produce Swap: Use pears instead of apples for a fall-inspired twist.
Dietary Substitutions: Omit the honey for a lower-sugar option.

DESSERTS

DESSERTS

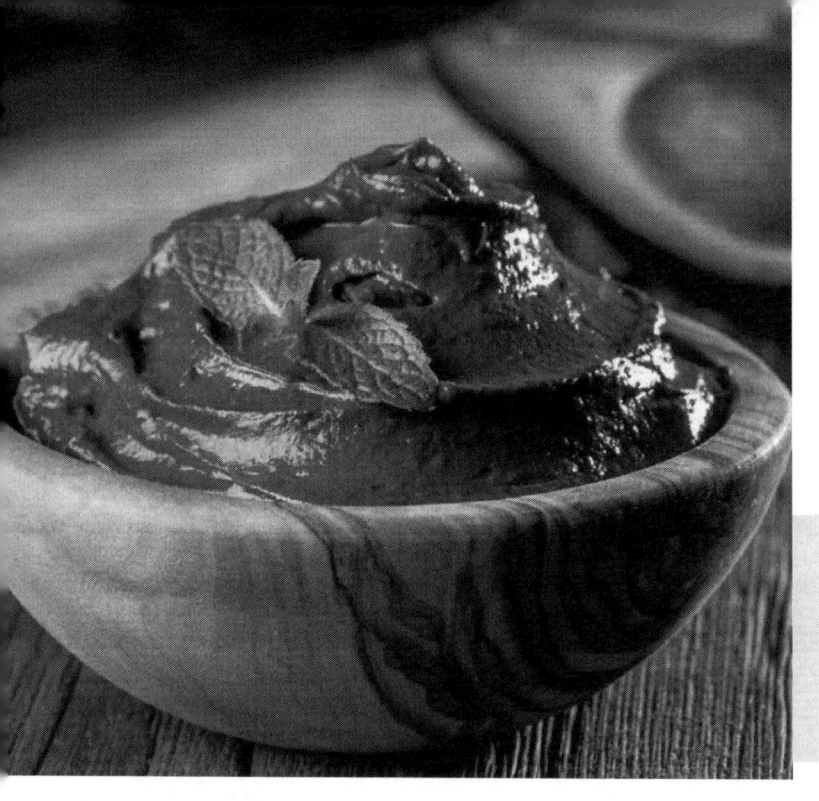

DARK CHOCOLATE AVOCADO MOUSSE

Anti-Inflammatory Benefits:
Avocados provide healthy monounsaturated fats, while dark chocolate is rich in antioxidants and flavonoids that combat inflammation.

PREP TIME: 10 MINS

COOK TIME: 00 MINS

SERVING: 3
Portion Size: 1 small bowl per serving

INGREDIENTS

- 1 ripe avocado (200 g), peeled and pitted
- 1/4 cup (25 g) unsweetened cocoa powder
- 3 tbsp (45 ml) maple syrup
- 1/4 cup (60 ml) almond milk
- 1/2 tsp (2.5 ml) vanilla extract

EQUIPMENT NEEDED:
Blender or food processor, mixing bowl

INSTRUCTIONS

1. Place the avocado, cocoa powder, maple syrup, almond milk, and vanilla extract in a food blender.
2. Blend on full power until the ingredient's texture looks smooth and creamy, scraping down the sides as needed.
3. Spoon the mousse into small wide-mouth bowls and chill for 15 minutes before serving.

NUTRITIONAL INFORMATION (PER SERVING):

Calories: 180 kcal, Carbohydrates: 18 g, Protein: 3 g, Fat: 12 g, Fiber: 5 g

HEALTH BENEFITS:
Seasonal Produce Swap: Add fresh berries or sliced bananas as a topping.
Dietary Substitutions: Use agave syrup instead of maple syrup for a lighter flavor.

DESSERTS

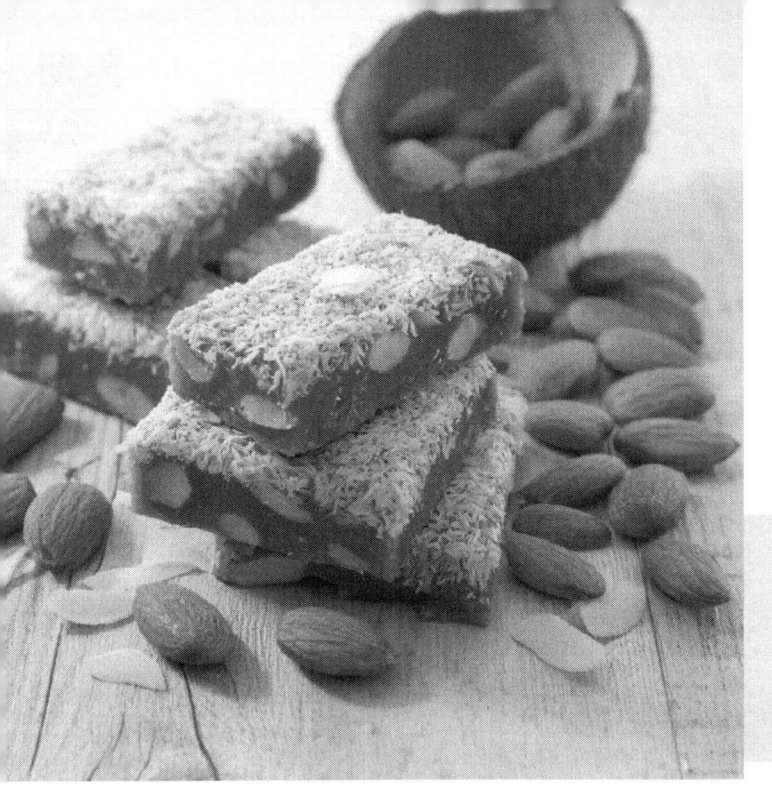

COCONUT AND ALMOND ENERGY BARS

Anti-Inflammatory Benefits:
Coconut and almonds are rich in healthy fats, while dates provide natural sweetness and antioxidants.

PREP TIME: 10 MINS

COOK TIME: 00 MINS

SERVING: 6
Portion Size: 2 bars per serving

INGREDIENTS

- 1 cup (100 g) almonds
- 1/2 cup (50 g) shredded unsweetened coconut
- 6 dates (120 g), pitted
- 1 tbsp (15 ml) coconut oil
- 1/2 tsp (2.5 ml) vanilla extract

EQUIPMENT NEEDED:
Food processor, baking dish

INSTRUCTIONS

1. Place the almonds, shredded coconut, dates, coconut oil, and vanilla extract in a food processor.
2. Blend on full power until the mixture turns into sticky dough.
3. Press the mixture into the parchment paper-arranged baking dish lined with parchment paper.
4. Refrigerate for 30 minutes, then cut into bars and serve.

NUTRITIONAL INFORMATION (PER SERVING):

Calories: 210 kcal, Carbohydrates: 15 g, Protein: 4 g, Fat: 16 g, Fiber: 4 g

HEALTH BENEFITS:
Seasonal Produce Swap: Add dried cranberries or apricots for variation.
Dietary Substitutions: Replace almonds with sunflower seeds for a nut-free version.

DESSERTS

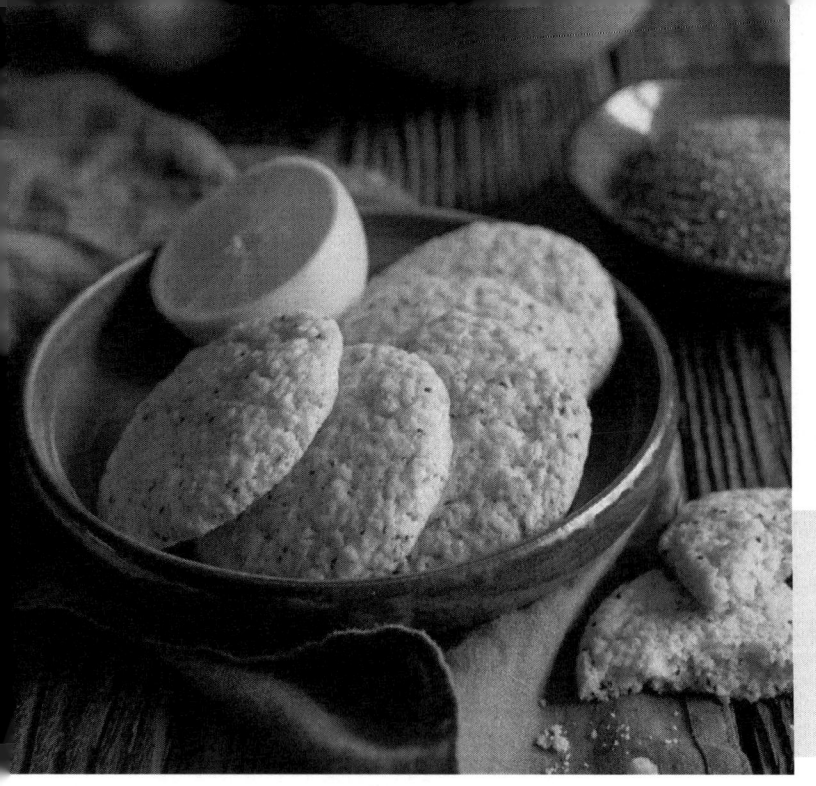

LEMON AND CHIA SEED COOKIES

Anti-Inflammatory Benefits:
Lemon provides vitamin C, while chia seeds are a source of omega-3 fatty acids that help reduce inflammation.

PREP TIME: 10 MINS
COOK TIME: 12 MINS
SERVING: 12 Portion Size: 3 cookies per serving

INGREDIENTS

- 1 cup (120 g) almond flour
- 2 tbsp (15 g) chia seeds
- 2 tbsp (30 ml) maple syrup
- 1 tbsp (15 ml) lemon juice
- 1/2 tsp (2.5 ml) vanilla extract

EQUIPMENT NEEDED:
Blender or food processor, mixing bowl

INSTRUCTIONS

1. Preheat oven to 350°F (175°C). Arrange the baking sheet with parchment paper.
2. Take a large, deep-bottom bowl and combine almond flour, chia seeds, maple syrup, lemon juice, and vanilla extract. Mix until a dough forms.
3. Scoop fully loaded tablespoon portions of dough onto the baking sheet and flatten slightly.
4. Bake for 10–12 minutes until the edges look golden. Let cool before serving.

NUTRITIONAL INFORMATION (PER SERVING):

Calories: 150 kcal, Carbohydrates: 10 g, Protein: 3 g, Fat: 10 g, Fiber: 3 g

HEALTH BENEFITS:
Seasonal Produce Swap: Use orange juice and zest for a different citrus flavor.
Dietary Substitutions: Replace almond flour with oat flour for a nut-free option.

DESSERTS

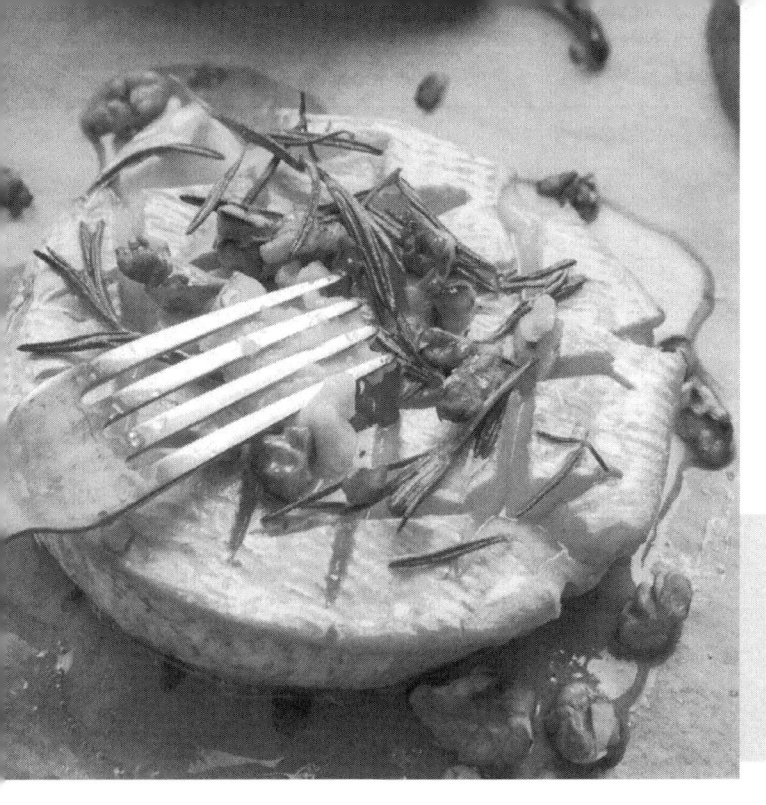

BAKED PEARS WITH WALNUTS AND HONEY

Anti-Inflammatory Benefits:
Pears are rich in fiber and antioxidants, while walnuts provide omega-3 fatty acids, and honey has natural anti-inflammatory properties.

PREP TIME: 5 MINS

COOK TIME: 15 MINS

SERVING: 2
Portion Size: 1 baked pear per serving

INGREDIENTS

- 2 medium pears (300 g), halved and cored
- 1/4 cup (30 g) walnuts, chopped
- 1 tbsp (15 ml) honey

EQUIPMENT NEEDED:
Baking dish, spoon

INSTRUCTIONS

1. Preheat oven to 375°F (190°C).
2. Place the pear halves in the parchment paper-arranged baking dish. Fill the center of each pear with chopped walnuts.
3. Drizzle with sweetener (honey or any other) and bake for 15 minutes or until tender.
4. Serve warm as a simple, healthy dessert.

NUTRITIONAL INFORMATION (PER SERVING):

Calories: 150 kcal, Carbohydrates: 25 g, Protein: 2 g, Fat: 6 g, Fiber: 5 g

HEALTH BENEFITS:
Seasonal Produce Swap: Use apples instead of pears for variety.
Dietary Substitutions: Replace honey with maple syrup for a vegan option.

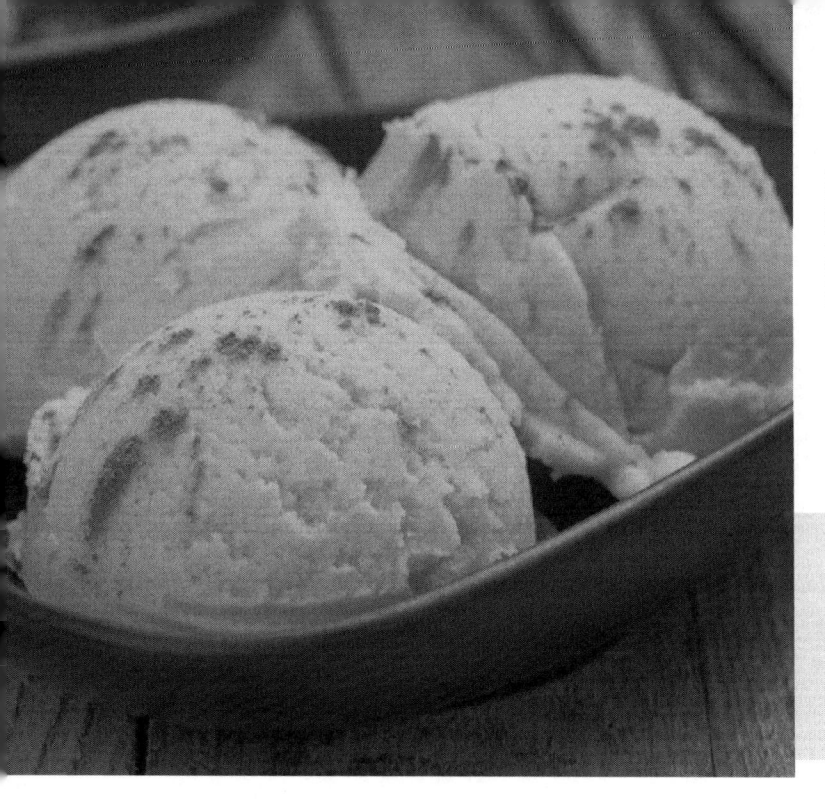

MATCHA GREEN TEA ICE CREAM

DESSERTS

Anti-Inflammatory Benefits:
Matcha is rich in antioxidants, particularly catechins, which combat inflammation and support overall health.

PREP TIME: 10 MINS
COOK TIME: 00 MINS
SERVING: 4
Portion Size: 1 small bowl per serving

INGREDIENTS

- 1 can (400 ml) coconut milk
- 2 tbsp (10 g) matcha green tea powder
- 1/4 cup (60 ml) maple syrup
- 1/2 tsp (2.5 ml) vanilla extract

EQUIPMENT NEEDED:
Blender, freezer-safe container

INSTRUCTIONS

1. Blend coconut milk, matcha powder, maple syrup, and vanilla extract in a blender until smooth.
2. Ladle the mixture into the container (should be freezer-safe) and freeze for 2–3 hours, stirring every 30 minutes to prevent ice crystals.
3. Scoop into bowls and serve immediately.

NUTRITIONAL INFORMATION (PER SERVING):

Calories: 180 kcal, Carbohydrates: 15 g, Protein: 2 g, Fat: 14 g, Fiber: 1 g

HEALTH BENEFITS:
Seasonal Produce Swap: Top with fresh berries for a fruity twist.
Dietary Substitutions: Use almond milk instead of coconut milk for a lighter option.

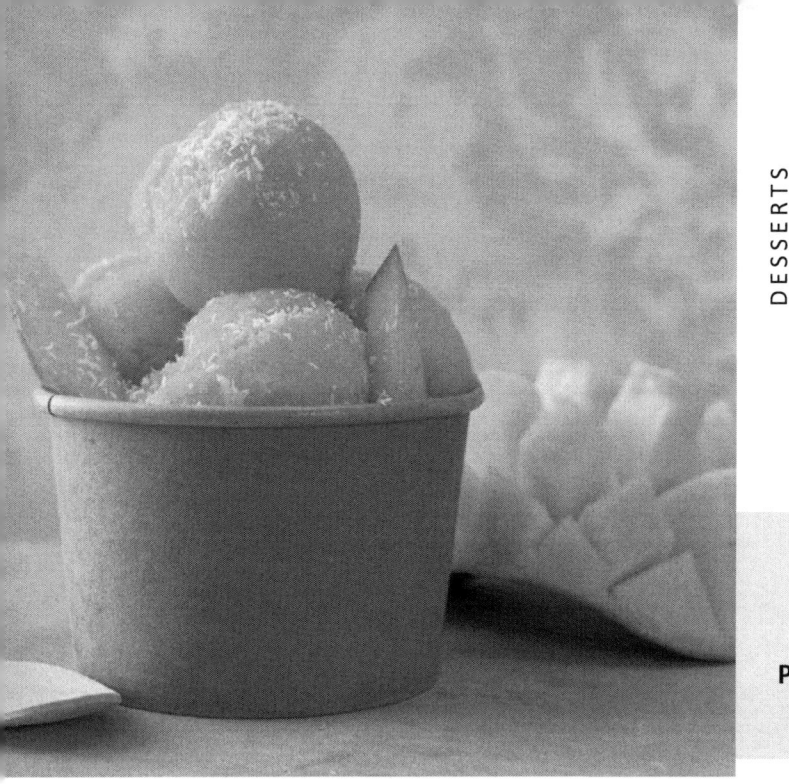

MANGO COCONUT SORBET

DESSERTS

Anti-Inflammatory Benefits:
Mangoes are high in vitamin C and antioxidants, while coconut milk provides healthy fats to reduce inflammation.

PREP TIME: 5 MINS

COOK TIME: 00 MINS

SERVING: 3
Portion Size: 1 small bowl per serving

INGREDIENTS

- 2 cups (300 g) frozen mango chunks
- 1/2 cup (120 ml) coconut milk
- 1 tbsp (15 ml) lime juice

INSTRUCTIONS

1. Blend mango chunks, coconut milk, and lime juice in a blender until smooth.
2. Pour into a freezer-safe container and freeze for 2 hours.
3. Scoop into bowls and serve cold.

EQUIPMENT NEEDED:
Blender, freezer-safe container

NUTRITIONAL INFORMATION (PER SERVING):

Calories: 130 kcal, Carbohydrates: 22 g, Protein: 1 g, Fat: 4 g, Fiber: 2 g

HEALTH BENEFITS:
Seasonal Produce Swap: Use peaches or pineapples instead of mangoes.
Dietary Substitutions: Add a splash of orange juice for a citrusy flavor.

DESSERTS

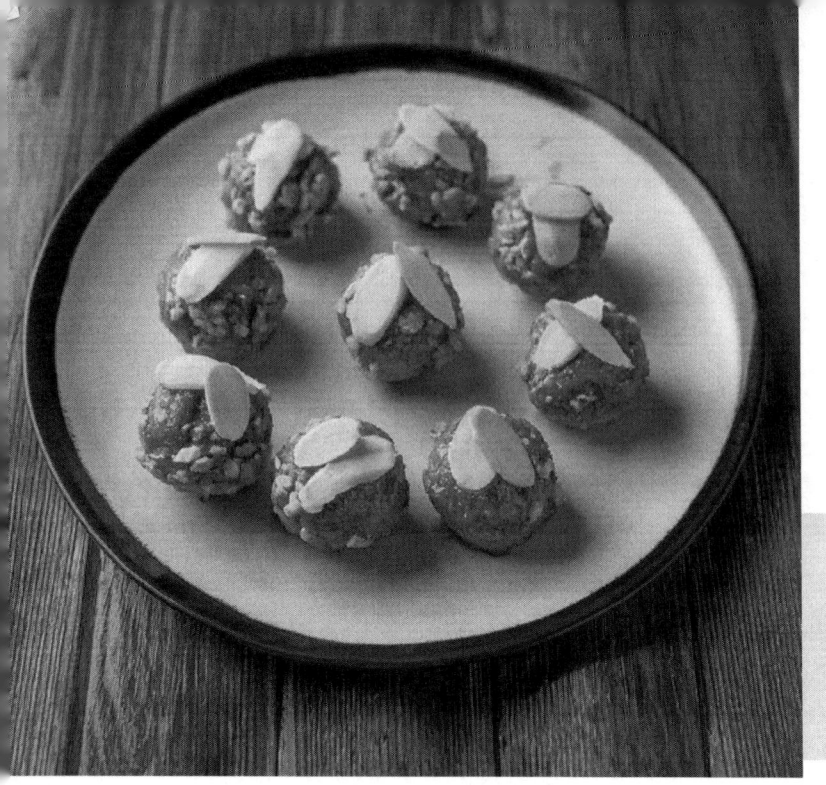

BANANA AND ALMOND BUTTER BITES

Anti-Inflammatory Benefits:
Bananas are rich in potassium, while almond butter provides vitamin E and healthy fats that reduce inflammation.

PREP TIME: 5 MINS
COOK TIME: 00 MINS
SERVING: 3
Portion Size: 5 bites per serving

INGREDIENTS

- 2 medium bananas (200 g), sliced into rounds
- 1/4 cup (60 g) almond butter

EQUIPMENT NEEDED:
Knife, parchment paper

INSTRUCTIONS

1. Spread almond butter onto half of the banana slices.
2. Top with the remaining slices to form "banana sandwiches."
3. Place on a parchment-lined tray and freeze for 1 hour.
4. Serve frozen as a quick and satisfying snack.

NUTRITIONAL INFORMATION (PER SERVING):

Calories: 150 kcal, Carbohydrates: 20 g, Protein: 4 g, Fat: 6 g, Fiber: 3 g

HEALTH BENEFITS:
Seasonal Produce Swap: Use sliced apples or pears instead of bananas.
Dietary Substitutions: Replace almond butter with sunflower seed butter for a nut-free version.

DESSERTS

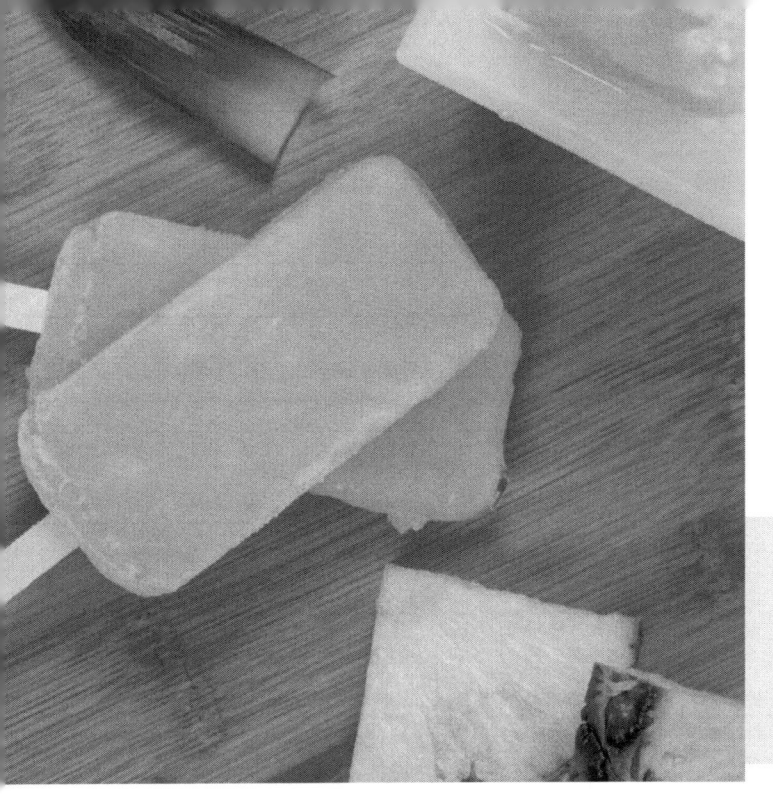

PINEAPPLE AND GINGER POPSICLES

Anti-Inflammatory Benefits:
Pineapple contains bromelain, a natural anti-inflammatory enzyme, while ginger supports digestion and reduces inflammation.

PREP TIME: 5 MINS

COOK TIME: 00 MINS

SERVING: 6
Portion Size: 2 popsicles per serving

INGREDIENTS

- 2 cups (300 g) fresh pineapple chunks
- 1/2 tsp (1 g) grated ginger
- 1/2 cup (120 ml) coconut water

EQUIPMENT NEEDED:
Blender, popsicle molds

INSTRUCTIONS

1. Blend pineapple, ginger, and coconut water in a blender until smooth.
2. Ladle mixture into popsicle molds and freeze for 4 hours (at least) until solid.
3. Remove from molds and serve frozen.

NUTRITIONAL INFORMATION (PER SERVING):

Calories: 80 kcal, Carbohydrates: 18 g, Protein: 0 g, Fat: 0 g, Fiber: 2 g

HEALTH BENEFITS:

Seasonal Produce Swap: Use watermelon or cantaloupe for a summer variation.
Dietary Substitutions: Add a splash of lime juice for extra zest.

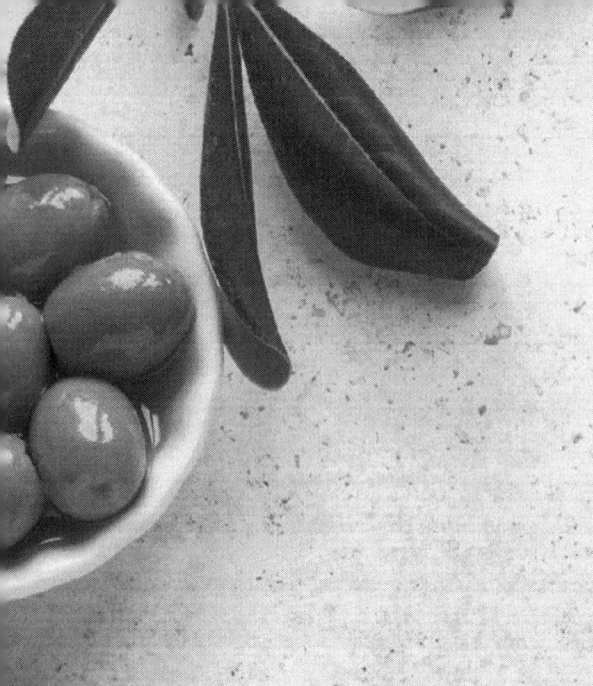

CONCLUSION

As you reach the end of Everyday Anti-Inflammatory Diet Cookbook: 100 Simple Recipes to Reduce Inflammation, Boost Immunity, and Feel Your Best, I hope you feel inspired and empowered to embrace the healing power of food. This book isn't just a collection of recipes—it's a tool to help you nurture your body, prioritize your health, and make cooking a joyful part of your daily life.

By incorporating these anti-inflammatory meals into your routine, you're taking meaningful steps toward reducing inflammation, boosting immunity, and enhancing your overall well-being. Whether it's through the vibrant colors of fresh vegetables, the comforting warmth of a nourishing soup, or the indulgent sweetness of a wholesome dessert, these recipes are here to support you on your journey to better health.

Remember, wellness isn't about perfection—it's about consistency and balance. Small, sustainable changes to your eating habits can make a profound impact over time. Celebrate your progress, explore new flavors, and enjoy the process of fueling your body with foods that make you feel your best.

Thank you for letting this cookbook be part of your wellness journey. I hope it brings you not only delicious meals but also a deeper connection to your health and the joy of cooking. Here's to a life filled with vibrant flavors, good health, and happiness—one bite at a time.

Printed in Great Britain
by Amazon